PRACTICAL COLOR ATLAS
OF
SECTIONAL ANATOMY

PRACTICAL COLOR ATLAS OF SECTIONAL ANATOMY

Chest, Abdomen, and Pelvis

E. A. Lyons, MD, FRCP(C), FACR

Director of Diagnostic Ultrasound
Health Sciences Centre
Professor of Radiology and Lecturer in Anatomy
University of Manitoba
Winnipeg, Manitoba, Canada

RAVEN PRESS 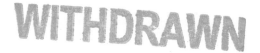 NEW YORK

Raven Press, 1185 Avenue of the Americas, New York, New York 10036

Printed and bound in Hong Kong

Library of Congress Cataloging-in-Publication Data
Lyons, Edward A. (Edward Arthur), 1943–
    Practical color atlas of sectional anatomy : chest, abdomen, and pelvis / E.A. Lyons.
        p.   cm.
    Rev. ed of: A color atlas of sectional anatomy.   1978.
    Includes index.
    ISBN 0-88167-550-4
    1. Chest—Atlases.   2. Abdomen—Atlases.   3. Pelvis—Atlases.
I. Lyons, Edward A. (Edward Arthur).   1943–   Color atlas of
sectional anatomy.   II. Title.
    [DNLM: 1. Abdomen—anatomy & histology—atlases. 2. Pelvis—
anatomy & histology—atlases.   3. Thorax—anatomy & histology—
atlases.   WE 17 L991c]
QM540.L95   1989
611'.9—dc20
DNLM/DLC
for Library of Congress   89–8400
                                                                    CIP

The material contained in this volume was submitted as previously unpublished material, except in the instances in which credit has been given to the source from which some of the illustrative material was derived.

Great care has been taken to maintain the accuracy of the information contained in the volume. However, neither Raven Press nor the editors can be held responsible for errors or for any consequences arising from the use of the information contained herein.

Materials appearing in this book prepared by individuals as part of their official duties as U.S. Government employees are not covered by the above-mentioned copyright.

9   8   7   6   5   4   3   2   1

To my family

Harriet

Mara

and

Sami

Preface

This atlas represents a revision of the original published in 1978. Several changes were made to add additional labeling and to reduce the physical size of the work, making it more affordable and easier to use.

Sectional imaging is now a routine part of our diagnostic lives. Ultrasound, computed tomography (CT), magnetic resonance imaging (MRI), radio-isotope studies such as single photon emission computed tomography (SPECT), positron emission tomography (PET), and X-ray tomography all view the body in "slices" through various anatomical planes.

Imaging specialists must understand sectional anatomy. All medical practitioners who use the information gleaned from these many imaging procedures should also be familiar with sectional anatomy in order to "interpret" the reported findings of the imaging specialist. As these images pervade all general and specialty medical journals, it should provide additional incentive to become familiar with these new techniques. Finally, all medical students MUST learn sectional anatomy as well as the standard anatomical presentations so that they will be prepared for "the view" that lies ahead.

E. A. Lyons

Acknowledgments

As with every undertaking, there are a number of people whose contributions must be acknowledged, for without their presence the task would have been more difficult, if not impossible.

My parents provided the initial stimulus in my medical career, especially my father, also a physician. He established a high personal standard in his own field of obstetrics, which he continues to maintain after 40 years of practice. My goals are to achieve, in some small measure, some of his professional fulfillment. It was on his insistence that I spent my summers of undergraduate medical training in research, which led directly to my career in ultrasound and to this anatomical undertaking.

The late Dr. M. G. Saunders was my first mentor in ultrasound and was followed by Dr. Ross E. Brown and Prof. I. Donald. I am grateful for their early guidance. Dr. D. W. MacEwan, professor of radiology, has been a continuous source of encouragement.

The book began as a means of teaching sectional anatomy to my staff and students. Their day-to-day stimulation and inquisitiveness provided the impetus to continue. My thanks to Shael Harris, Darrel Barkman, Kathy McDiarmid, Denis Gratton, Bruce Goalen, Gene Charney, Gerry Ballard, Julie Hay, and Doug Shaw.

My colleagues in the Department of Anatomy at the University of Manitoba—Dr. K. Moore, Dr. R. E. Grahame, and Dr. T. V. Persaud—assisted me in every way, and without their complete cooperation this book would not have been possible.

The technical aspect of preparing and sectioning the cadavers fell to Syd Bradbury and Ray St. Hilaire. Their willingness to assist and their expertise have been much appreciated. We were fortunate enough to be able to utilize the facilities of the Provincial Veterinary Lab, for which I am truly grateful.

The sections were photographed by Rob Mathieson, a master at his craft. He did an outstanding job in capturing the color and detail of the original sections. I was also fortunate to have the support of the Department of Medical Photography at the Health Sciences Centre as a whole and of its director, Ken McGregor, in particular.

All of the art work was done by David Lee, who did an admirable job on all of the line diagrams.

In the arduous task of labeling all pertinent structures, I received tremendous assistance and support from Dr. Ruvin Lyons and Dr. R. E. Grahame. I am indebted to them for their help.

Finally, for the thread that held the whole thing together—my wife, Har—words cannot express my gratitude.

E. A. Lyons

Contents

Introduction

The purpose of this atlas is to portray normal anatomy and anatomical relationships as simply as possible. To accomplish this, serial sections 1 cm thick were prepared using frozen cadavers not previously embalmed. The major arterial and venous systems were injected with red and blue latex solutions respectively. Each section can therefore be presented in such a way as to preserve the natural color of all the organs with some artificial accentuation of the vascular tree. In addition to the use of color as an aid to rapid identification, a large number of sections are presented in a serial fashion so as to provide a sense of continuity as well as for the sake of completeness. Using this kind of presentation, I have tried to present as detailed an atlas as possible. It was not feasible to identify some of the small yet significant structures in each and every section. In such instances, it is hoped that the reader will refer to the sections before and after the one of interest to find the structure in question. If one remembers that each section is only 1 cm thick, the relative position of all structures should be satisfactorily locatable. Every attempt has been made to be honest, so that where a structure could not accurately be identified, its label was omitted from that section but may be found in subsequent ones.

Sections were cut in the three major anatomical planes: *transverse* or *cross* sections, *parasagittal* or *longitudinal* sections, and *coronal* sections. Again, to provide a continuum of sections, the general layout of the book emphasizes the *plane of sections* rather than the general anatomical region. For example, transverse sections of the chest, abdomen, and pelvis are presented one after the other. This was most important for the transverse plane where the chest and abdominal sections were from the same cadaver. A definite continuity is maintained throughout the body.

Part One   TRANSVERSE SECTIONS

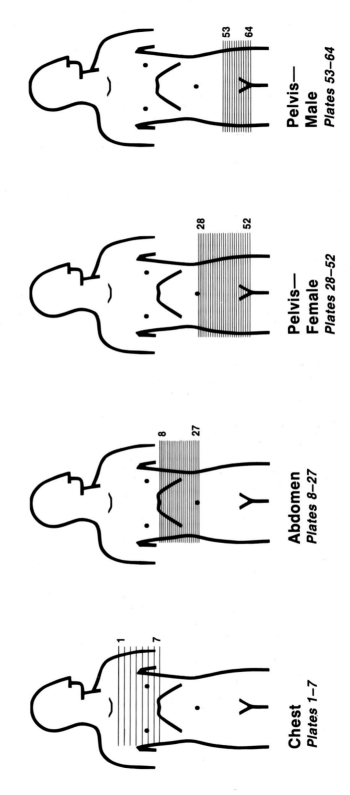

Chest
Plates 1–7

Abdomen
Plates 8–27

**Pelvis—
Female**
Plates 28–52

**Pelvis—
Male**
Plates 53–64

TRANSVERSE Chest *Plates 1–7*

Plate 1

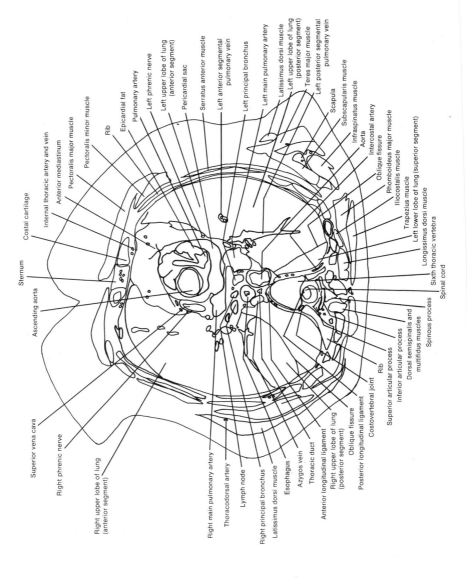

Superior vena cava
Right phrenic nerve
Right upper lobe of lung (anterior segment)

Right main pulmonary artery
Thoracodorsal artery
Lymph node
Right principal bronchus
Latissimus dorsi muscle
Esophagus
Azygos vein
Thoracic duct
Anterior longitudinal ligament
Right upper lobe of lung (posterior segment)
Oblique fissure
Posterior longitudinal ligament
Costovertebral joint
Rib
Superior articular process
Inferior articular process
Dorsal semispinalis and multifidus muscles
Spinous process

Sternum
Costal cartilage
Internal thoracic artery and vein
Anterior mediastinum
Pectoralis major muscle
Pectoralis minor muscle
Rib
Epicardial fat
Pulmonary artery
Left phrenic nerve
Left upper lobe of lung (anterior segment)
Pericardial sac
Serratus anterior muscle
Left anterior segmental pulmonary vein
Left principal bronchus

Ascending aorta

Left main pulmonary artery
Latissimus dorsi muscle
Left upper lobe of lung (posterior segment)
Teres major muscle
Left posterior segmental pulmonary vein
Scapula
Subscapularis muscle
Infraspinatus muscle
Aorta
Intercostal artery
Oblique fissure
Rhomboideus major muscle
Iliocostalis muscle
Trapezius muscle
Left lower lobe of lung (superior segment)
Longissimus dorsi muscle
Sixth thoracic vertebra
Spinal cord

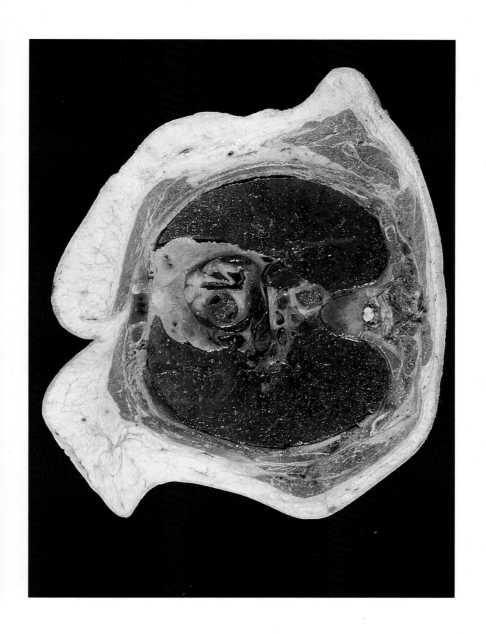

Plate 2

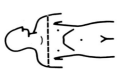

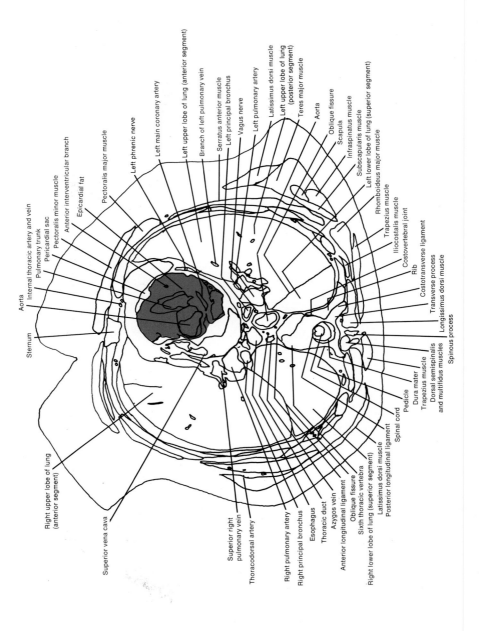

Aorta
Internal thoracic artery and vein
Pulmonary trunk
Pericardial sac
Pectoralis minor muscle
Anterior interventricular branch
Epicardial fat
Pectoralis major muscle
Left phrenic nerve
Left main coronary artery
Left upper lobe of lung (anterior segment)
Branch of left pulmonary vein
Serratus anterior muscle
Left principal bronchus
Vagus nerve
Left pulmonary artery
Left upper lobe of lung (posterior segment)
Latissimus dorsi muscle
Teres major muscle
Aorta
Oblique fissure
Scapula
Infraspinatus muscle
Subscapularis muscle
Left lower lobe of lung (superior segment)
Rhomboideus major muscle
Trapezius muscle
Iliocostalis muscle
Costovertebral joint
Rib
Costotransverse ligament
Transverse process
Longissimus dorsi muscle
Spinous process
Dorsal semispinalis and multifidus muscles
Dura mater
Pedicle
Spinal cord
Trapezius muscle
Posterior longitudinal ligament
Latissimus dorsi muscle
Right lower lobe of lung (superior segment)
Sixth thoracic vertebra
Oblique fissure
Anterior longitudinal ligament
Azygos vein
Thoracic duct
Esophagus
Right principal bronchus
Right pulmonary artery
Thoracodorsal artery
Superior right pulmonary vein
Right upper lobe of lung (anterior segment)
Superior vena cava
Sternum

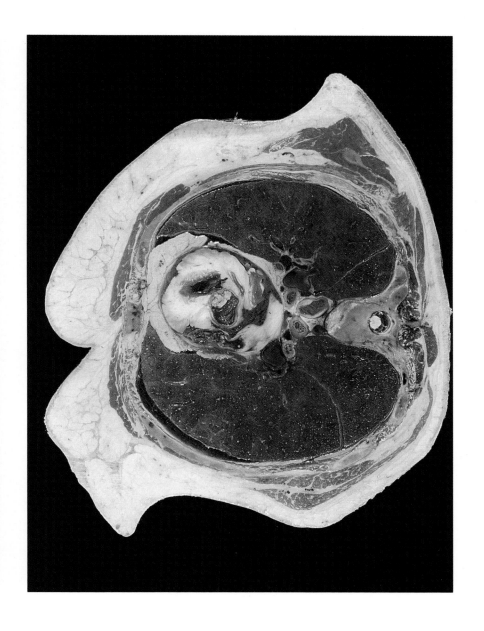

Plate 3

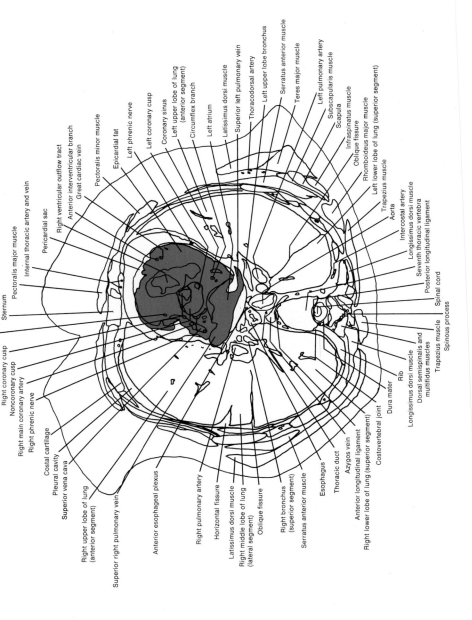

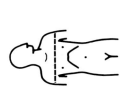

Right coronary artery
Right coronary cusp
Noncoronary cusp
Right main coronary artery
Right phrenic nerve
Costal cartilage
Pleural cavity
Superior vena cava

Superior right pulmonary vein

Anterior esophageal plexus

Right pulmonary artery

Horizontal fissure
Latissimus dorsi muscle
Right middle lobe of lung
(lateral segment)
Oblique fissure

Right upper lobe of lung
(anterior segment)

Right bronchus
(superior segment)
Serratus anterior muscle

Esophagus

Thoracic duct

Azygos vein

Anterior longitudinal ligament

Right lower lobe of lung (superior segment)

Costovertebral joint

Dura mater

Longissimus dorsi muscle

Rib

Longissimus dorsi muscle
Dorsal semispinalis and
multifidus muscles

Trapezius muscle
Spinous process

Pectoralis major muscle
Internal thoracic artery and vein
Pericardial sac
Right ventricular outflow tract
Anterior interventricular branch
Great cardiac vein
Pectoralis minor muscle
Epicardial fat
Left phrenic nerve
Left coronary cusp
Coronary sinus
Left upper lobe of lung
(anterior segment)
Circumflex branch
Left atrium
Latissimus dorsi muscle
Superior left pulmonary vein
Thoracodorsal artery
Left upper lobe bronchus
Serratus anterior muscle
Teres major muscle
Left pulmonary artery
Subscapularis muscle
Scapula
Infraspinatus muscle
Rhomboideus major muscle
Oblique fissure
Left lower lobe of lung (superior segment)
Trapezius muscle
Aorta
Intercostal artery
Longissimus dorsi muscle
Seventh thoracic vertebra
Posterior longitudinal ligament
Spinal cord
Sternum

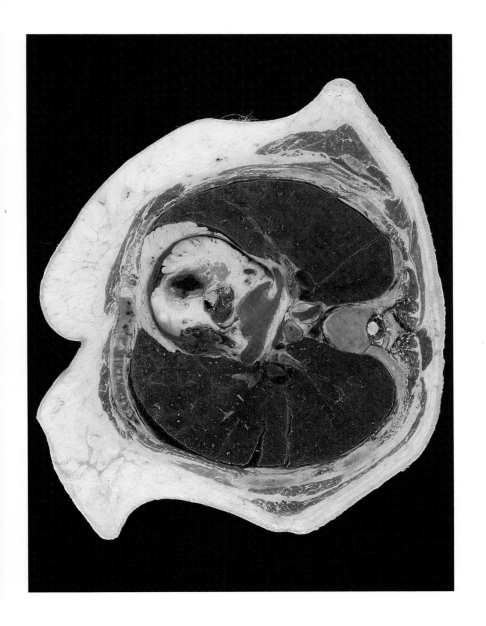

Transverse **Chest**

Plate 4

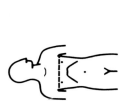

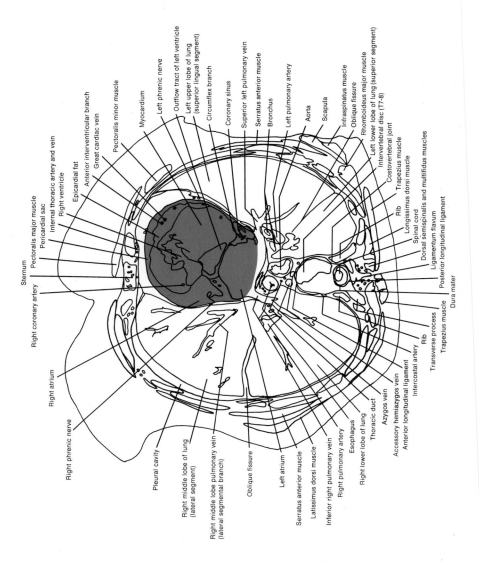

Sternum

Pectoralis major muscle

Pectoralis minor muscle

Internal thoracic artery and vein

Epicardial fat

Right ventricle

Anterior interventricular branch

Great cardiac vein

Myocardium

Left phrenic nerve

Outflow tract of left ventricle

Left upper lobe of lung (superior lingual segment)

Circumflex branch

Coronary sinus

Superior left pulmonary vein

Serratus anterior muscle

Bronchus

Left pulmonary artery

Aorta

Scapula

Infraspinatus muscle

Oblique fissure

Left lower lobe of lung (superior segment)

Rhomboideus major muscle

Intervertebral disc (T7-8)

Costovertebral joint

Trapezius muscle

Rib

Longissimus dorsi muscle

Spinal cord

Dorsal semispinalis and multifidus muscles

Ligamentum flavum

Posterior longitudinal ligament

Dura mater

Pericardial sac

Right coronary artery

Right atrium

Right phrenic nerve

Pleural cavity

Right middle lobe of lung (lateral segment)

Right middle lobe pulmonary vein (lateral segmental branch)

Oblique fissure

Left atrium

Serratus anterior muscle

Latissimus dorsi muscle

Inferior right pulmonary vein

Right pulmonary artery

Esophagus

Right lower lobe of lung

Thoracic duct

Azygos vein

Accessory hemiazygos vein

Anterior longitudinal ligament

Intercostal artery

Rib

Transverse process

Trapezius muscle

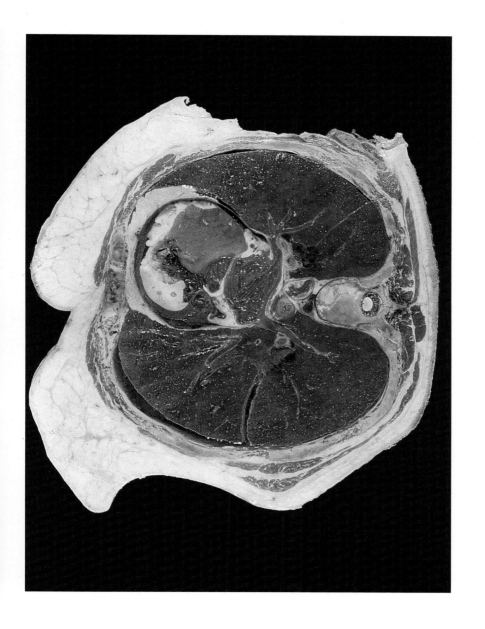

Transverse **Chest**

Plate 5

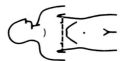

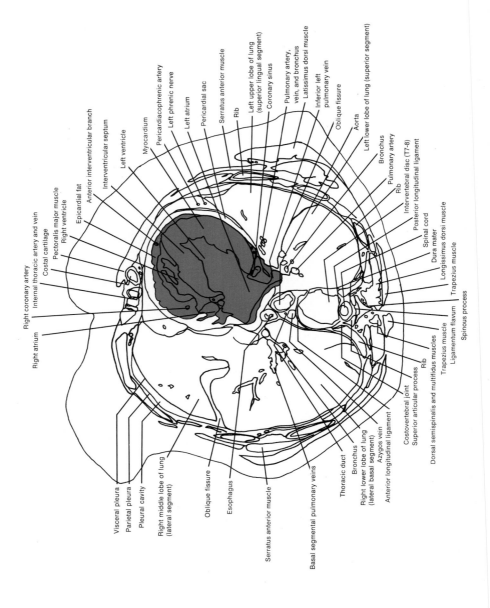

Right coronary artery
Internal thoracic artery and vein
Costal cartilage
Pectoralis major muscle
Right ventricle
Epicardial fat
Anterior interventricular branch
Interventricular septum
Left ventricle
Myocardium
Pericardiacophrenic artery
Left phrenic nerve
Left atrium
Pericardial sac
Serratus anterior muscle
Rib
Left upper lobe of lung (superior lingual segment)
Coronary sinus
Pulmonary artery, vein, and bronchus
Latissimus dorsi muscle
Inferior left pulmonary vein
Oblique fissure
Aorta
Left lower lobe of lung (superior segment)
Bronchus
Pulmonary artery
Rib
Intervertebral disc (T7-8)
Posterior longitudinal ligament
Spinal cord
Dura mater
Longissimus dorsi muscle
Trapezius muscle
Spinous process
Trapezius muscle
Ligamentum flavum
Rib
Dorsal semispinalis and multifidus muscles
Superior articular process
Costovertebral joint
Anterior longitudinal ligament
Azygos vein
Right lower lobe of lung (lateral basal segment)
Bronchus
Thoracic duct
Basal segmental pulmonary veins
Serratus anterior muscle
Esophagus
Oblique fissure
Right middle lobe of lung (lateral segment)
Pleural cavity
Parietal pleura
Visceral pleura
Right atrium

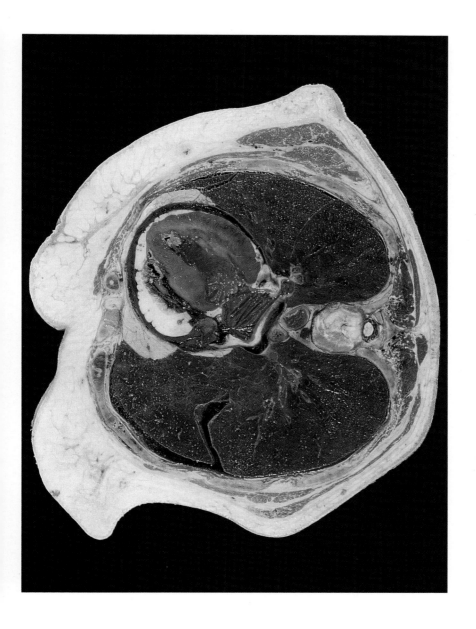

Transverse **Chest**

Plate 6

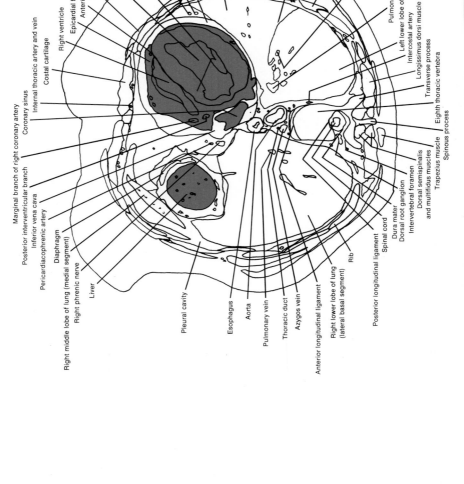

Marginal branch of right coronary artery
Posterior interventricular branch
Inferior vena cava
Pericardiacophrenic artery
Diaphragm
Right middle lobe of lung (medial segment)
Right phrenic nerve
Liver

Coronary sinus
Internal thoracic artery and vein
Costal cartilage
Right ventricle
Epicardial fat
Anterior interventricular branch
Pectoralis major muscle
Left ventricle
Interventricular septum
Pericardiacophrenic artery
Left phrenic nerve
Pericardial sac
Rib
Left upper lobe of lung (inferior lingular segment)
Thoracodorsal artery
Serratus anterior muscle
Oblique fissure
Latissimus dorsi muscle
Intercostal muscles
Pulmonary artery (segmental branch)
Pulmonary vein
Left lower lobe of lung (posterior basal segment)
Intercostal artery
Longissimus dorsi muscle
Transverse process
Eighth thoracic vertebra
Spinous process
Trapezius muscle
Dorsal semispinalis and multifidus muscles
Intervertebral foramen
Dorsal root ganglion
Dura mater
Spinal cord
Posterior longitudinal ligament
Rib
Right lower lobe of lung (lateral basal segment)
Anterior longitudinal ligament
Azygos vein
Thoracic duct
Pulmonary vein
Aorta
Esophagus
Pleural cavity

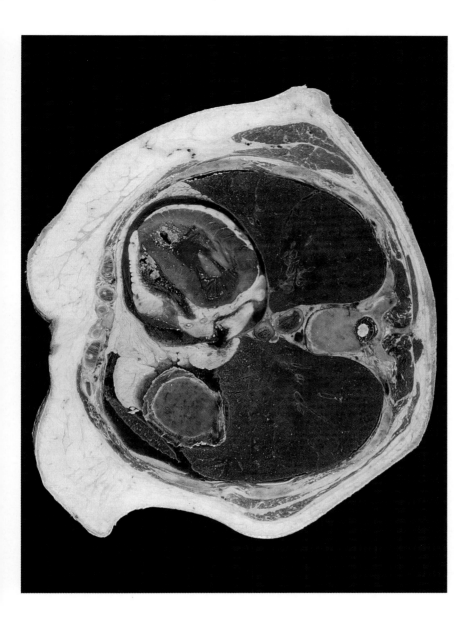

Transverse **Chest**

Plate 7

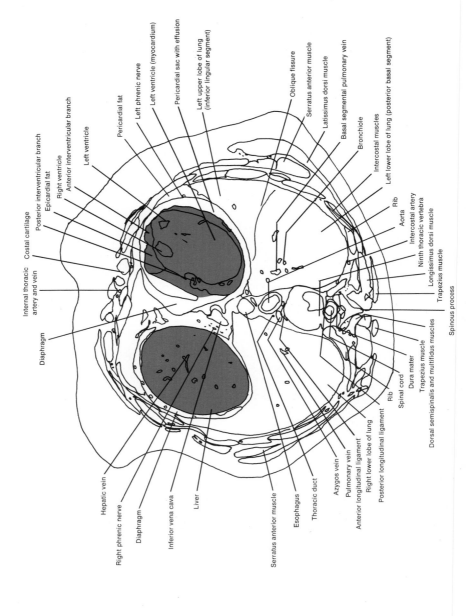

Internal thoracic
artery and vein

Costal cartilage

Posterior interventricular branch

Epicardial fat

Right ventricle

Anterior interventricular branch

Left ventricle

Pericardial fat

Left phrenic nerve

Left ventricle (myocardium)

Pericardial sac with effusion

Left upper lobe of lung
(inferior lingular segment)

Oblique fissure

Serratus anterior muscle

Latissimus dorsi muscle

Basal segmental pulmonary vein

Bronchiole

Intercostal muscles

Left lower lobe of lung (posterior basal segment)

Rib

Aorta

Intercostal artery

Ninth thoracic vertebra

Longissimus dorsi muscle

Trapezius muscle

Spinous process

Trapezius muscle

Dorsal semispinalis and multifidus muscles

Dura mater

Spinal cord

Rib

Posterior longitudinal ligament

Right lower lobe of lung

Anterior longitudinal ligament

Pulmonary vein

Azygos vein

Thoracic duct

Esophagus

Serratus anterior muscle

Liver

Inferior vena cava

Diaphragm

Right phrenic nerve

Hepatic vein

Diaphragm

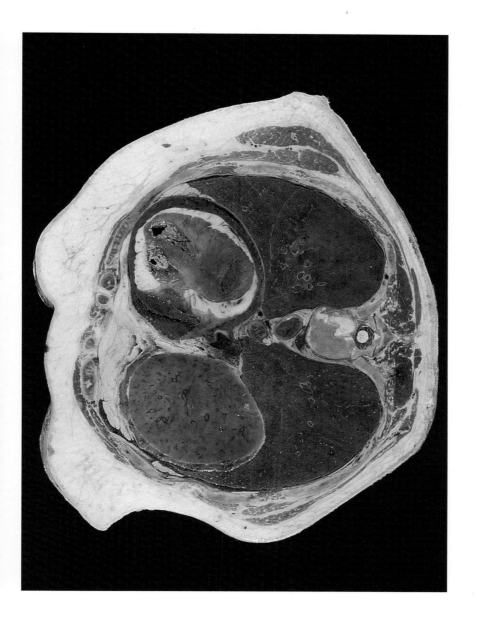

TRANSVERSE   Abdomen   *Plates 8–27*

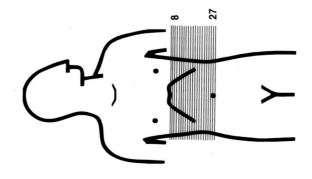

Renal Anatomy

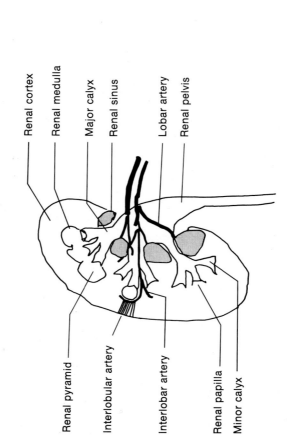

Renal cortex
Renal medulla
Major calyx
Renal sinus
Lobar artery
Renal pelvis

Renal pyramid
Interlobular artery
Interlobar artery
Renal papilla
Minor calyx

Plate 8

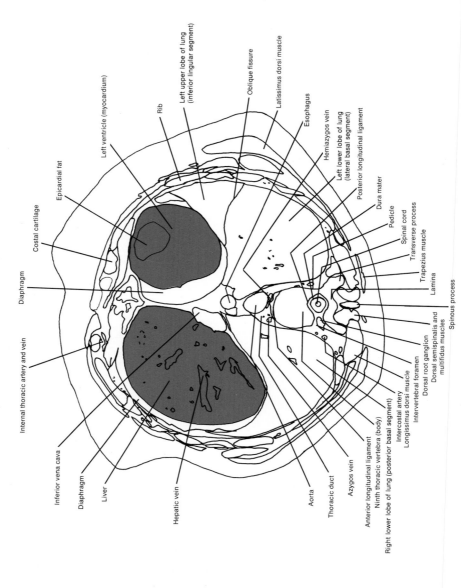

Inferior vena cava

Diaphragm

Liver

Hepatic vein

Right lower lobe of lung (posterior basal segment)

Ninth thoracic vertebra (body)

Anterior longitudinal ligament

Azygos vein

Thoracic duct

Aorta

Internal thoracic artery and vein

Diaphragm

Costal cartilage

Epicardial fat

Left ventricle (myocardium)

Rib

Left upper lobe of lung (inferior lingular segment)

Oblique fissure

Latissimus dorsi muscle

Esophagus

Hemiazygos vein

Left lower lobe of lung (lateral basal segment)

Posterior longitudinal ligament

Dura mater

Pedicle

Spinal cord

Transverse process

Trapezius muscle

Lamina

Spinous process

Dorsal semispinalis and multifidus muscles

Dorsal root ganglion

Intervertebral foramen

Longissimus dorsi muscle

Intercostal artery

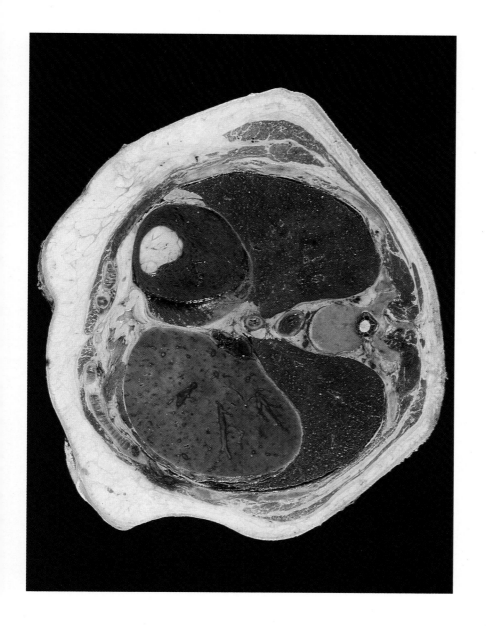

Transverse **Abdomen**

23

Plate 9

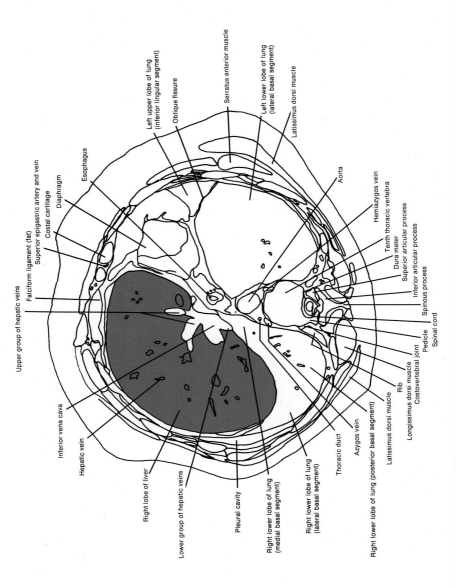

Upper group of hepatic veins

Falciform ligament (fat)
Superior epigastric artery and vein
Costal cartilage
Diaphragm
Esophagus

Left upper lobe of lung (inferior lingular segment)
Oblique fissure

Serratus anterior muscle

Left lower lobe of lung (lateral basal segment)

Latissimus dorsi muscle

Aorta

Hemiazygos vein

Tenth thoracic vertebra

Dura mater
Superior articular process
Inferior articular process
Spinous process
Pedicle
Spinal cord

Costovertebral joint

Rib

Longissimus dorsi muscle

Latissimus dorsi muscle

Azygos vein

Thoracic duct

Right lower lobe of lung (lateral basal segment)

Right lower lobe of lung (posterior basal segment)

Right lower lobe of lung (medial basal segment)

Pleural cavity

Lower group of hepatic veins

Right lobe of liver

Hepatic vein

Inferior vena cava

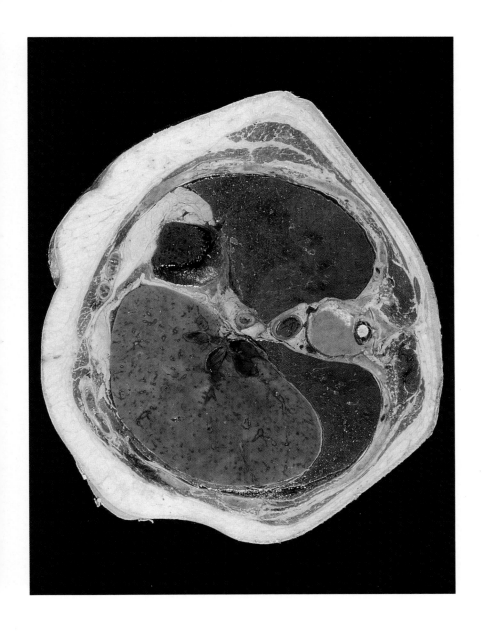

25

Transverse **Abdomen**

Plate 10

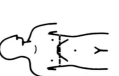

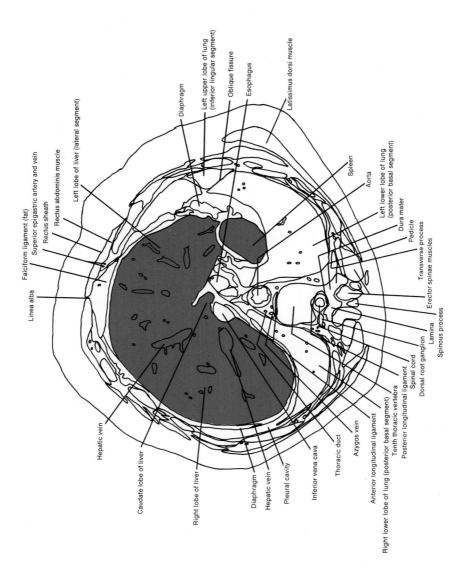

Diaphragm

Left upper lobe of lung (inferior lingular segment)

Oblique fissure

Esophagus

Latissimus dorsi muscle

Left lobe of liver (lateral segment)

Rectus abdominis muscle

Superior epigastric artery and vein

Rectus sheath

Falciform ligament (fat)

Linea alba

Spleen

Aorta

Left lower lobe of lung (posterior basal segment)

Dura mater

Pedicle

Transverse process

Erector spinae muscles

Spinous process

Lamina

Dorsal root ganglion

Spinal cord

Posterior longitudinal ligament

Tenth thoracic vertebra

Right lower lobe of lung (posterior basal segment)

Anterior longitudinal ligament

Azygos vein

Thoracic duct

Inferior vena cava

Pleural cavity

Hepatic vein

Diaphragm

Right lobe of liver

Caudate lobe of liver

Hepatic vein

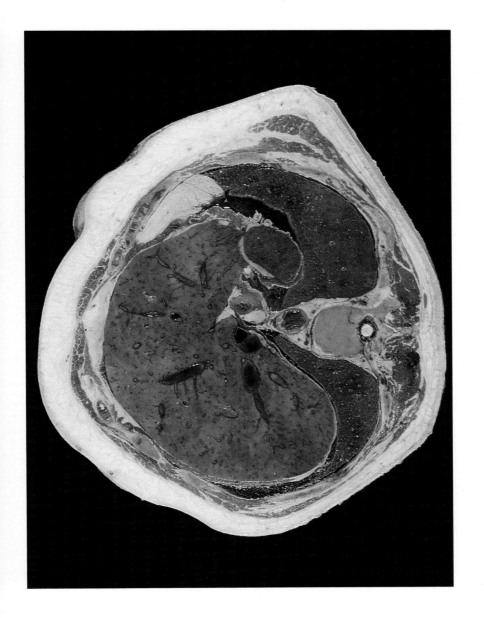

Transverse **Abdomen**

Plate 11

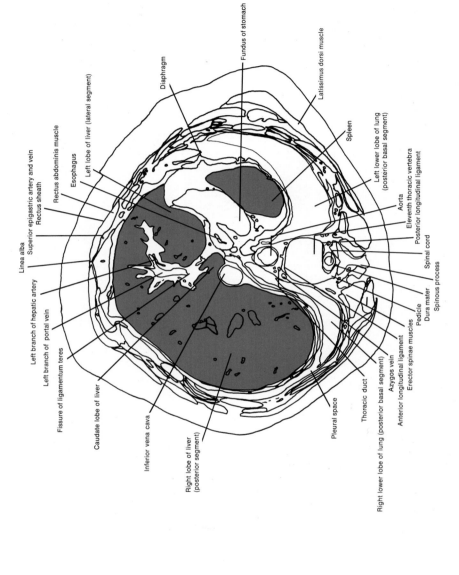

Fundus of stomach

Diaphragm

Left lobe of liver (lateral segment)

Esophagus

Rectus abdominis muscle

Rectus sheath

Superior epigastric artery and vein

Linea alba

Left branch of hepatic artery

Left branch of portal vein

Fissure of ligamentum teres

Caudate lobe of liver

Inferior vena cava

Right lobe of liver
(posterior segment)

Right lower lobe of lung (posterior basal segment)

Thoracic duct

Azygos vein

Anterior longitudinal ligament

Erector spinae muscles

Pleural space

Latissimus dorsi muscle

Spleen

Left lower lobe of lung
(posterior basal segment)

Aorta

Eleventh thoracic vertebra

Posterior longitudinal ligament

Spinal cord

Dura mater

Pedicle

Spinous process

29

Transverse **Abdomen**

Plate 12

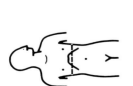

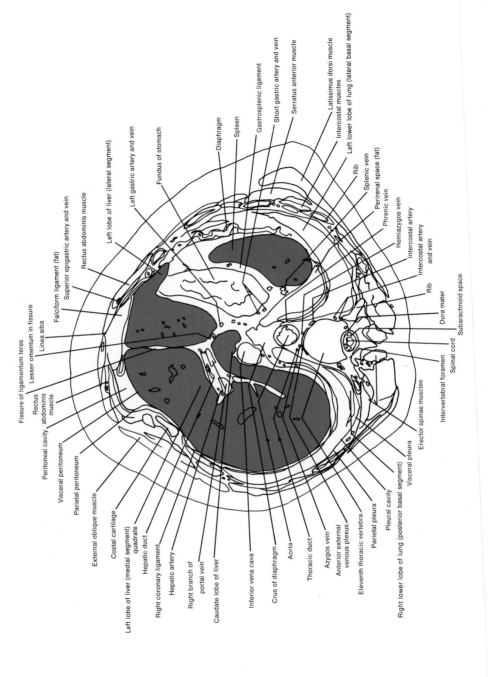

Fissure of ligamentum teres
Rectus
Lesser omentum in fissure
Rectus abdominis muscle
Peritoneal cavity,
Visceral peritoneum
Parietal peritoneum
External oblique muscle
Costal cartilage
Left lobe of liver (medial segment) quadrate
Hepatic duct
Right coronary ligament
Hepatic artery
Right branch of portal vein
Caudate lobe of liver
Inferior vena cava
Crus of diaphragm
Aorta
Thoracic duct
Azygos vein
Anterior external venous plexus
Eleventh thoracic vertebra
Right lower lobe of lung (posterior basal segment)
Pleural cavity
Parietal pleura
Visceral pleura
Erector spinae muscles
Intervertebral foramen
Spinal cord
Subarachnoid space
Dura mater
Rib
Intercostal artery and vein
Intercostal artery
Hemiazygos vein
Phrenic vein
Perirenal space (fat)
Splenic vein
Rib
Left lower lobe of lung (lateral basal segment)
Intercostal muscles
Latissimus dorsi muscle
Serratus anterior muscle
Short gastric artery and vein
Gastrosplenic ligament
Spleen
Diaphragm
Fundus of stomach
Left gastric artery and vein
Left lobe of liver (lateral segment)
Superior epigastric artery and vein
Falciform ligament (fat)
Linea alba
abdominis muscle

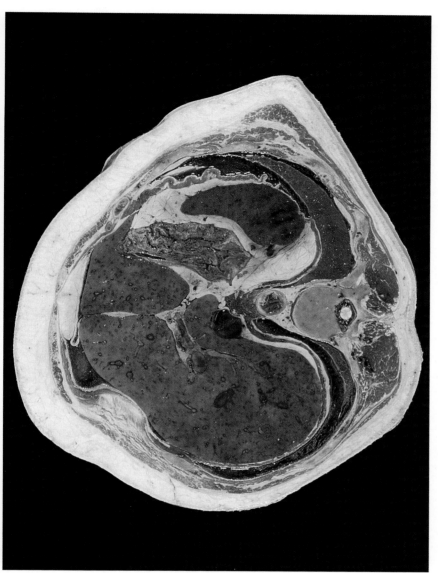

Transverse **Abdomen**

Plate 13

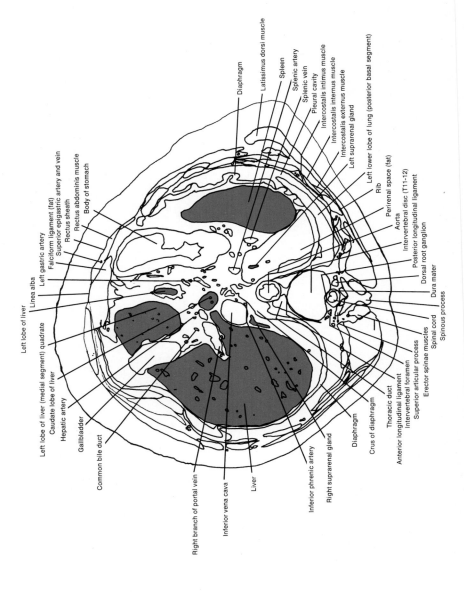

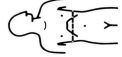

Left lobe of liver
Linea alba
Left lobe of liver (medial segment) quadrate
Caudate lobe of liver
Hepatic artery
Gallbladder
Common bile duct
Left gastric artery
Falciform ligament (fat)
Superior epigastric artery and vein
Rectus sheath
Rectus abdominis muscle
Body of stomach
Diaphragm
Latissimus dorsi muscle
Spleen
Splenic artery
Splenic vein
Pleural cavity
Intercostalis intimus muscle
Intercostalis internus muscle
Intercostalis externus muscle
Left suprarenal gland
Left lower lobe of lung (posterior basal segment)
Rib
Perirenal space (fat)
Aorta
Intervertebral disc (T11-12)
Posterior longitudinal ligament
Dorsal root ganglion
Dura mater
Spinous process
Spinal cord
Superior articular process
Intervertebral foramen
Anterior longitudinal ligament
Thoracic duct
Crus of diaphragm
Diaphragm
Right suprarenal gland
Inferior phrenic artery
Liver
Inferior vena cava
Right branch of portal vein
Erector spinae muscles

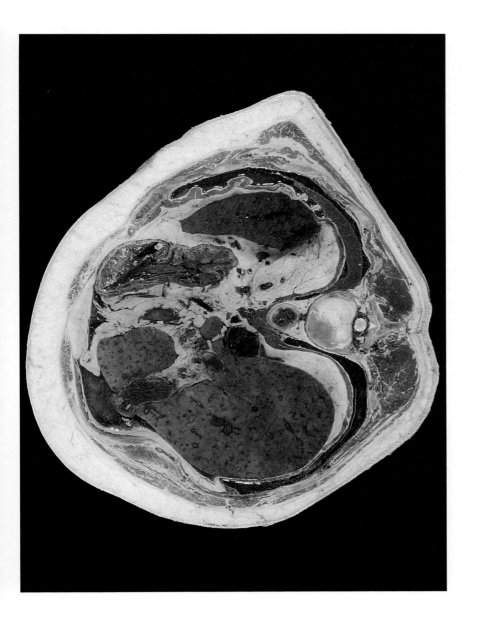

Transverse **Abdomen**

Plate 14

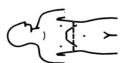

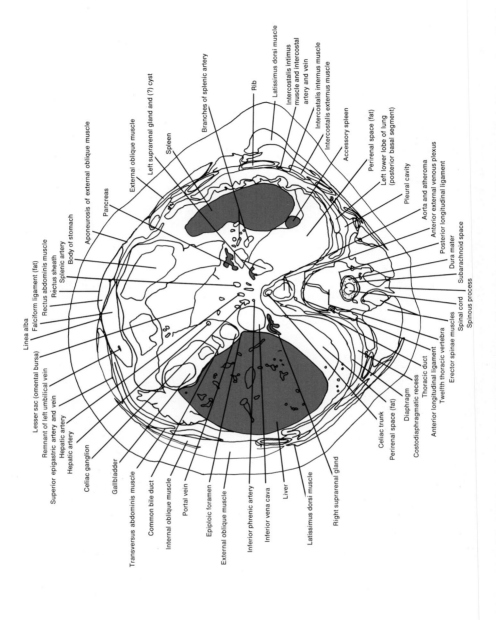

Linea alba
Falciform ligament (fat)
Lesser sac (omental bursa)
Remnant of left umbilical vein
Superior epigastric artery and vein
Hepatic artery and vein
Hepatic artery
Rectus abdominis muscle
Rectus sheath
Splenic artery
Body of stomach
Aponeurosis of external oblique muscle
Pancreas
External oblique muscle
Left suprarenal gland and (?) cyst
Spleen
Branches of splenic artery

Rib
Latissimus dorsi muscle
Intercostalis intimus muscle and intercostal artery and vein
Intercostalis internus muscle
Intercostalis externus muscle
Accessory spleen
Perirenal space (fat)
Left lower lobe of lung (posterior basal segment)
Pleural cavity
Aorta and atheroma
Anterior external venous plexus
Posterior longitudinal ligament
Dura mater
Subarachnoid space
Spinous process
Spinal cord
Erector spinae muscles
Twelfth thoracic vertebra
Anterior longitudinal ligament
Thoracic duct
Costodiaphragmatic recess
Diaphragm
Perirenal space (fat)
Celiac trunk
Right suprarenal gland
Latissimus dorsi muscle
Liver
Inferior vena cava
Inferior phrenic artery
External oblique muscle
Epiploic foramen
Portal vein
Internal oblique muscle
Common bile duct
Transversus abdominis muscle
Gallbladder
Celiac ganglion

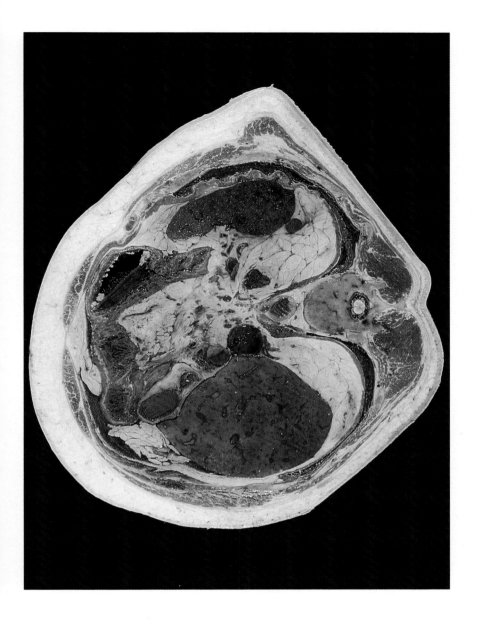

Transverse **Abdomen**

Plate 15

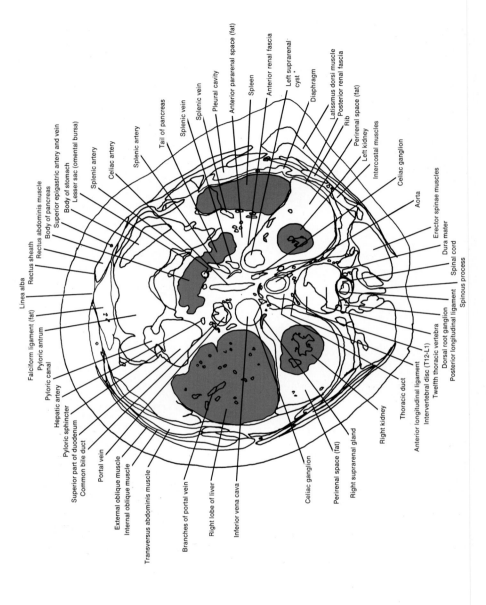

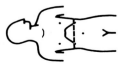

Linea alba
Falciform ligament (fat)
Rectus sheath
Pyloric antrum
Rectus abdominis muscle
Body of stomach
Pyloric canal
Body of pancreas
Superior epigastric artery and vein
Hepatic artery
Lesser sac (omental bursa)
Pyloric sphincter
Splenic artery
Superior part of duodenum
Celiac artery
Common bile duct
Splenic artery
Portal vein
Tail of pancreas
Splenic vein
Splenic vein
Pleural cavity
Anterior pararenal space (fat)
Anterior renal fascia
Spleen
Left suprarenal cyst *
Diaphragm
Latissimus dorsi muscle
Posterior renal fascia
Rib
Perirenal space (fat)
Left kidney
Intercostal muscles
Celiac ganglion
Aorta
Erector spinae muscles
Dura mater
Spinal cord
Spinous process
Posterior longitudinal ligament
Twelfth thoracic vertebra
Dorsal root ganglion
Intervertebral disc (T12-L1)
Anterior longitudinal ligament
Thoracic duct
Right kidney
Right suprarenal gland
Perirenal space (fat)
Celiac ganglion
Inferior vena cava
Right lobe of liver
Branches of portal vein
Transversus abdominis muscle
Internal oblique muscle
External oblique muscle

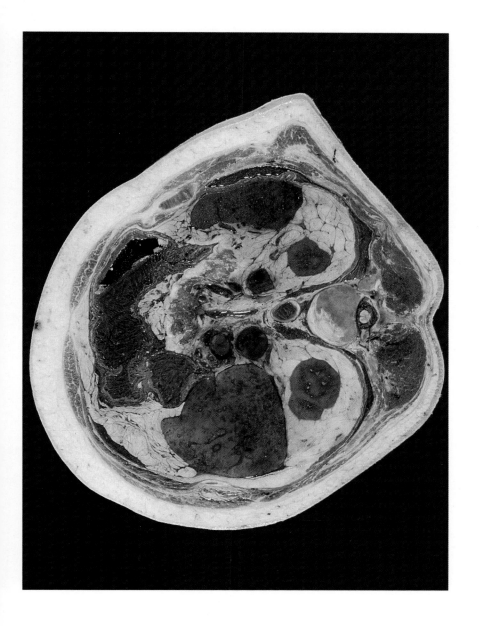

Transverse **Abdomen**

Plate 16

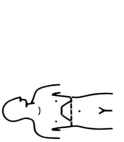

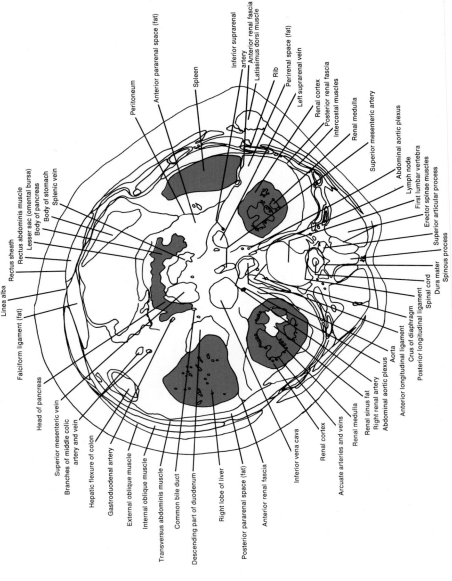

Linea alba
Rectus sheath
Rectus abdominis muscle
Lesser sac (omental bursa)
Body of pancreas
Body of stomach
Splenic vein

Peritoneum

Anterior pararenal space (fat)

Spleen

Inferior suprarenal artery
Anterior renal fascia
Latissimus dorsi muscle
Rib
Perirenal space (fat)
Left suprarenal vein

Renal cortex
Posterior renal fascia
Intercostal muscles

Renal medulla

Superior mesenteric artery

Abdominal aortic plexus

Lymph node

First lumbar vertebra

Erector spinae muscles

Superior articular process

Spinous process

Dura mater

Spinal cord

Posterior longitudinal ligament

Crus of diaphragm

Anterior longitudinal ligament

Aorta

Abdominal aortic plexus

Right renal artery

Renal sinus fat

Renal medulla

Arcuate arteries and veins

Renal cortex

Inferior vena cava

Anterior renal fascia

Posterior pararenal space (fat)

Right lobe of liver

Descending part of duodenum

Common bile duct

Transversus abdominis muscle

Internal oblique muscle

External oblique muscle

Gastroduodenal artery

Hepatic flexure of colon

Branches of middle colic artery and vein

Superior mesenteric vein

Head of pancreas

Falciform ligament (fat)

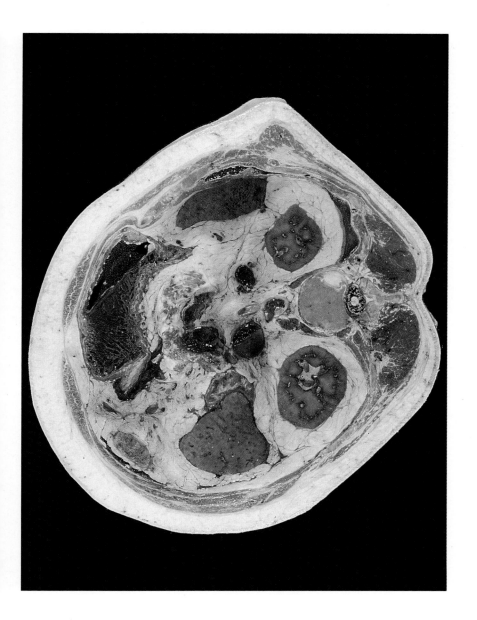

Transverse **Abdomen**

Plate 17

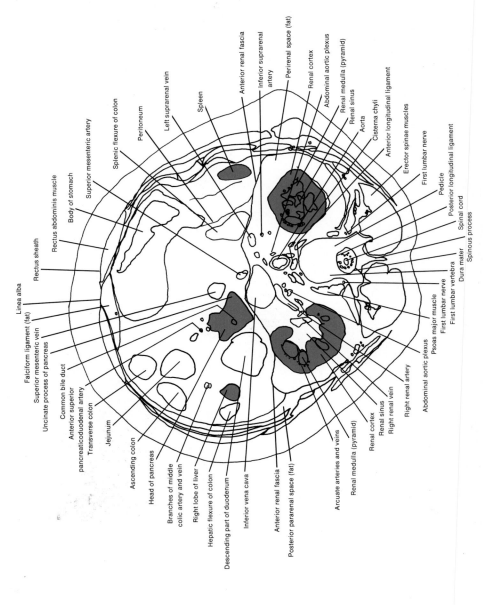

Transverse **Abdomen**

Plate 18

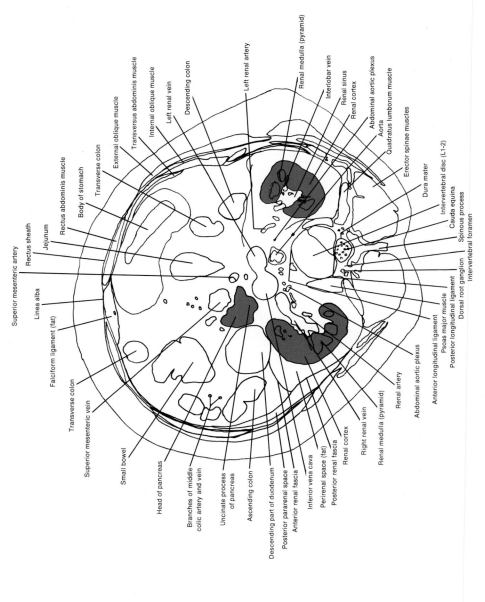

Superior mesenteric artery

Rectus sheath

Linea alba

Jejunum

Rectus abdominis muscle

Falciform ligament (fat)

Body of stomach

Transverse colon

External oblique muscle

Transversus abdominis muscle

Internal oblique muscle

Left renal vein

Descending colon

Left renal artery

Renal medulla (pyramid)

Interlobar vein

Renal sinus

Renal cortex

Abdominal aortic plexus

Aorta

Quadratus lumborum muscle

Erector spinae muscles

Dura mater

Intervertebral disc (L1-2)

Cauda equina

Spinous process

Intervertebral foramen

Dorsal root ganglion

Posterior longitudinal ligament

Psoas major muscle

Anterior longitudinal ligament

Abdominal aortic plexus

Renal artery

Renal medulla (pyramid)

Right renal vein

Renal cortex

Posterior renal fascia

Perirenal space (fat)

Inferior vena cava

Anterior renal fascia

Posterior pararenal space

Descending part of duodenum

Ascending colon

Uncinate process of pancreas

Branches of middle colic artery and vein

Head of pancreas

Small bowel

Superior mesenteric vein

Transverse colon

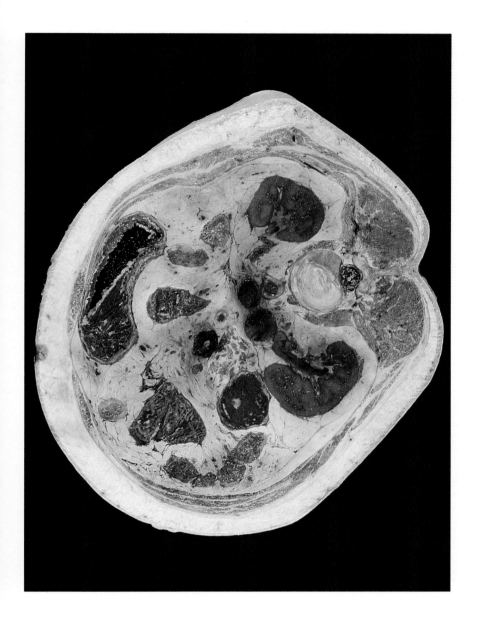

Transverse **Abdomen**

Plate 19

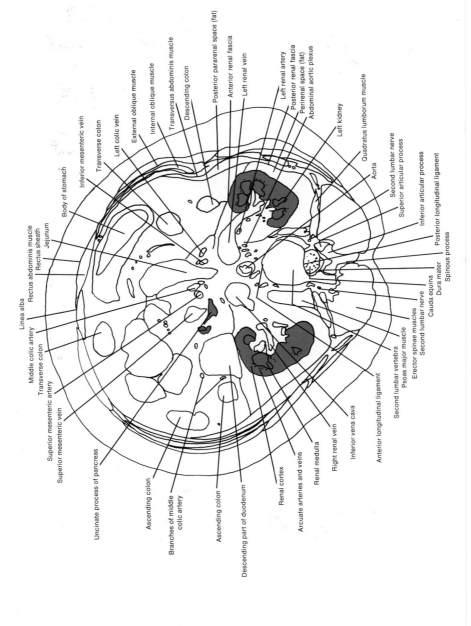

Linea alba
Middle colic artery
Transverse colon
Superior mesenteric artery
Superior mesenteric vein
Uncinate process of pancreas
Ascending colon
Branches of middle colic artery
Ascending colon
Descending part of duodenum
Renal cortex
Arcuate arteries and veins
Renal medulla
Right renal vein
Inferior vena cava
Anterior longitudinal ligament
Second lumbar vertebra
Psoas major muscle
Erector spinae muscles
Second lumbar nerve
Cauda equina
Dura mater
Second lumbar nerve
Posterior longitudinal ligament
Spinous process
Inferior articular process
Superior articular process
Aorta
Quadratus lumborum muscle
Left kidney
Abdominal aortic plexus
Perirenal space (fat)
Posterior renal fascia
Left renal artery
Left renal vein
Anterior renal fascia
Posterior pararenal space (fat)
Descending colon
Transversus abdominis muscle
Internal oblique muscle
External oblique muscle
Left colic vein
Transverse colon
Inferior mesenteric vein
Body of stomach
Jejunum
Rectus sheath
Rectus abdominis muscle

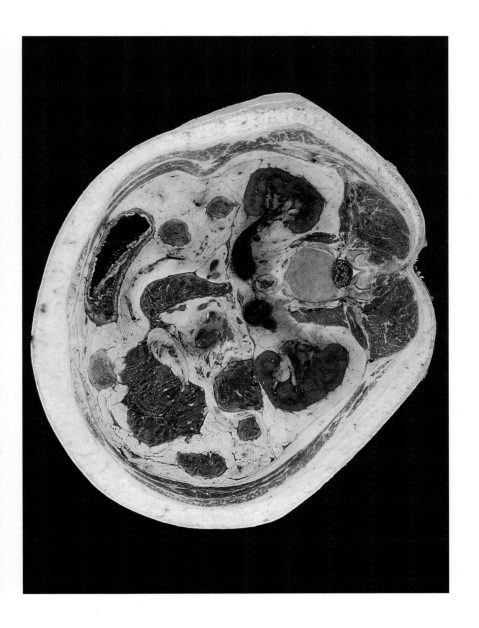

45

Transverse **Abdomen**

Plate 20

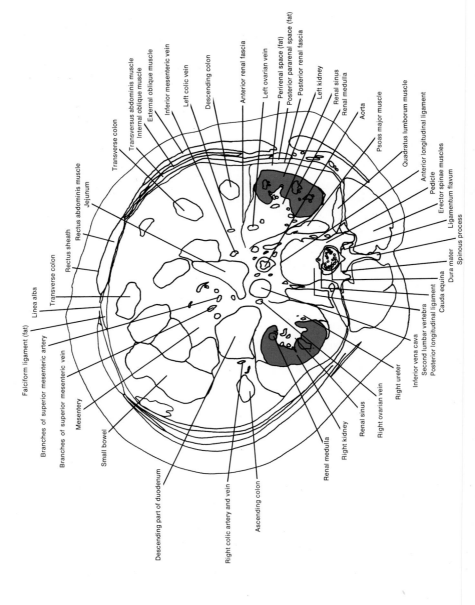

- Falciform ligament (fat)
- Linea alba
- Branches of superior mesenteric artery
- Transverse colon
- Branches of superior mesenteric vein
- Rectus sheath
- Mesentery
- Rectus abdominis muscle
- Jejunum
- Transverse colon
- Transversus abdominis muscle
- Internal oblique muscle
- External oblique muscle
- Inferior mesenteric vein
- Left colic vein
- Descending colon
- Anterior renal fascia
- Left ovarian vein
- Perirenal space (fat)
- Posterior pararenal space (fat)
- Posterior renal fascia
- Left kidney
- Renal sinus
- Renal medulla
- Aorta
- Psoas major muscle
- Quadratus lumborum muscle
- Anterior longitudinal ligament
- Erector spinae muscles
- Pedicle
- Ligamentum flavum
- Spinous process
- Dura mater
- Cauda equina
- Posterior longitudinal ligament
- Second lumbar vertebra
- Inferior vena cava
- Right ureter
- Right ovarian vein
- Renal sinus
- Right kidney
- Renal medulla
- Ascending colon
- Right colic artery and vein
- Descending part of duodenum
- Small bowel

Transverse **Abdomen**

Plate 21

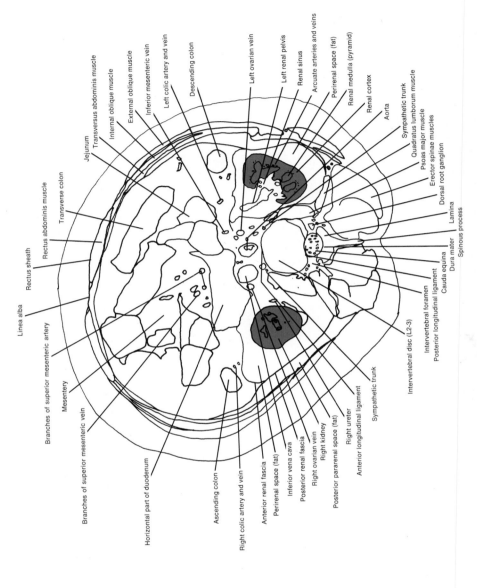

Linea alba

Rectus sheath

Rectus abdominis muscle

Transverse colon

Jejunum

Transversus abdominis muscle

Internal oblique muscle

External oblique muscle

Inferior mesenteric vein

Left colic artery and vein

Descending colon

Left ovarian vein

Left renal pelvis

Renal sinus

Arcuate arteries and veins

Perirenal space (fat)

Renal medulla (pyramid)

Renal cortex

Aorta

Sympathetic trunk

Quadratus lumborum muscle

Psoas major muscles

Erector spinae muscles

Dorsal root ganglion

Lamina

Spinous process

Dura mater

Cauda equina

Posterior longitudinal ligament

Intervertebral foramen

Intervertebral disc (L2-3)

Sympathetic trunk

Anterior longitudinal ligament

Right ureter

Posterior pararenal space (fat)

Right kidney

Right ovarian vein

Posterior renal fascia

Inferior vena cava

Perirenal space (fat)

Anterior renal fascia

Right colic artery and vein

Ascending colon

Horizontal part of duodenum

Branches of superior mesenteric vein

Mesentery

Branches of superior mesenteric artery

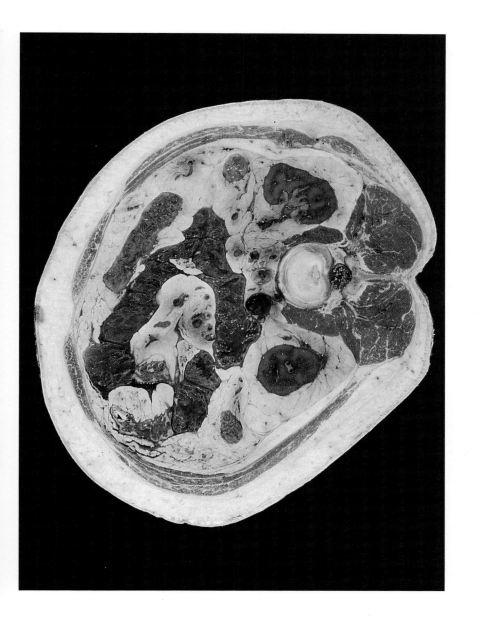

Transverse **Abdomen**

Plate 22

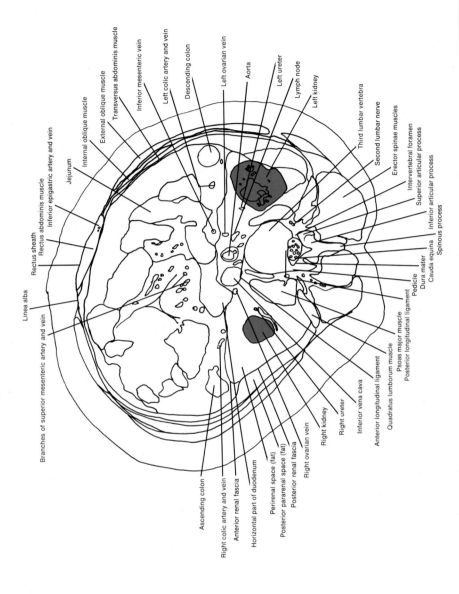

Linea alba

Rectus sheath

Inferior epigastric artery and vein

Rectus abdominis muscle

Jejunum

Internal oblique muscle

External oblique muscle

Transversus abdominis muscle

Inferior mesenteric vein

Left colic artery and vein

Descending colon

Left ovarian vein

Aorta

Left ureter

Lymph node

Left kidney

Third lumbar vertebra

Second lumbar nerve

Erector spinae muscles

Intervertebral foramen

Superior articular process

Inferior articular process

Spinous process

Cauda equina

Dura mater

Pedicle

Posterior longitudinal ligament

Psoas major muscle

Quadratus lumborum muscle

Anterior longitudinal ligament

Inferior vena cava

Right ureter

Right kidney

Right ovarian vein

Posterior renal fascia

Posterior pararenal space (fat)

Perirenal space (fat)

Horizontal part of duodenum

Anterior renal fascia

Right colic artery and vein

Ascending colon

Branches of superior mesenteric artery and vein

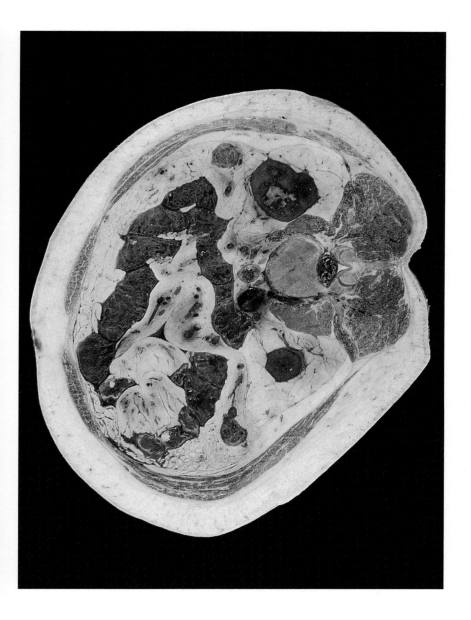

Transverse **Abdomen**

Plate 23

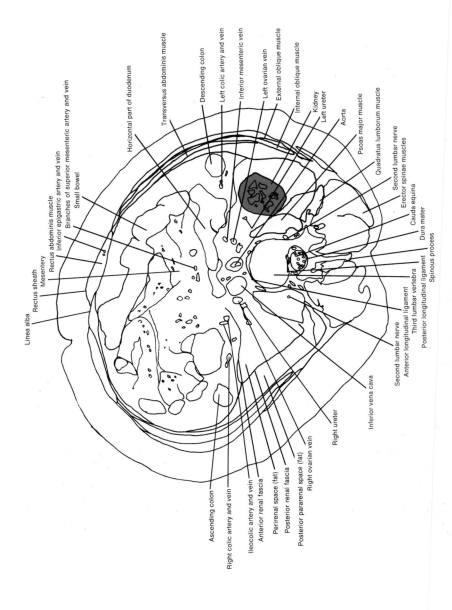

Linea alba
Rectus sheath
Mesentery
Rectus abdominis muscle
Inferior epigastric artery and vein
Branches of superior mesenteric artery and vein
Small bowel
Horizontal part of duodenum
Transversus abdominis muscle
Descending colon
Left colic artery and vein
Inferior mesenteric vein
Left ovarian vein
External oblique muscle
Internal oblique muscle
Kidney
Left ureter
Aorta
Psoas major muscle
Quadratus lumborum muscle
Second lumbar nerve
Erector spinae muscles
Cauda equina
Dura mater
Spinous process
Posterior longitudinal ligament
Third lumbar vertebra
Anterior longitudinal ligament
Second lumbar nerve
Inferior vena cava
Right ureter
Posterior pararenal space (fat)
Posterior renal fascia
Perirenal space (fat)
Anterior renal fascia
Ileocolic artery and vein
Right ovarian vein
Right colic artery and vein
Ascending colon

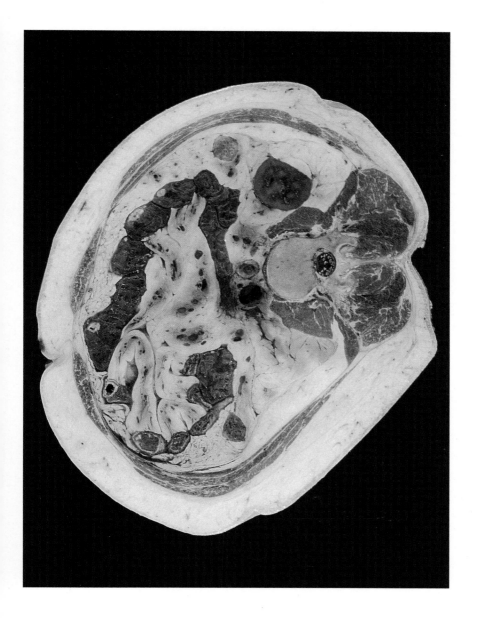

Plate 24

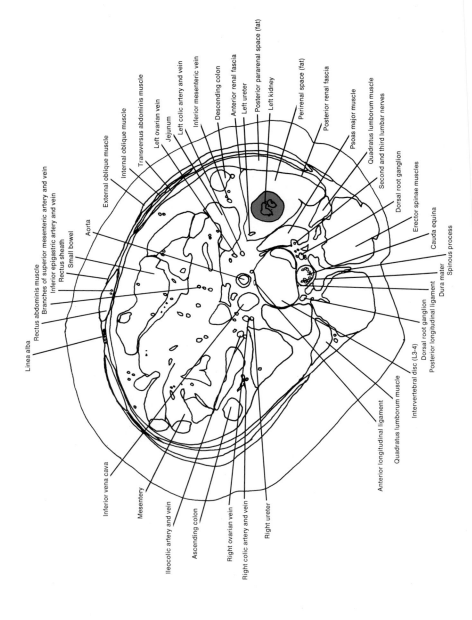

Linea alba
Rectus abdominis muscle
Branches of superior mesenteric artery and vein
Inferior epigastric artery and vein
Rectus sheath
Small bowel
Aorta

External oblique muscle
Internal oblique muscle
Transversus abdominis muscle
Left ovarian vein
Jejunum
Left colic artery and vein
Inferior mesenteric vein
Descending colon
Anterior renal fascia
Left ureter
Posterior pararenal space (fat)
Left kidney
Perirenal space (fat)
Posterior renal fascia
Psoas major muscle
Quadratus lumborum muscle
Second and third lumbar nerves
Dorsal root ganglion
Erector spinae muscles
Cauda equina
Spinous process
Dura mater
Posterior longitudinal ligament
Dorsal root ganglion
Intervertebral disc (L3-4)
Quadratus lumborum muscle
Anterior longitudinal ligament

Right ureter
Right colic artery and vein
Right ovarian vein
Ascending colon
Ileocolic artery and vein
Mesentery
Inferior vena cava

Y

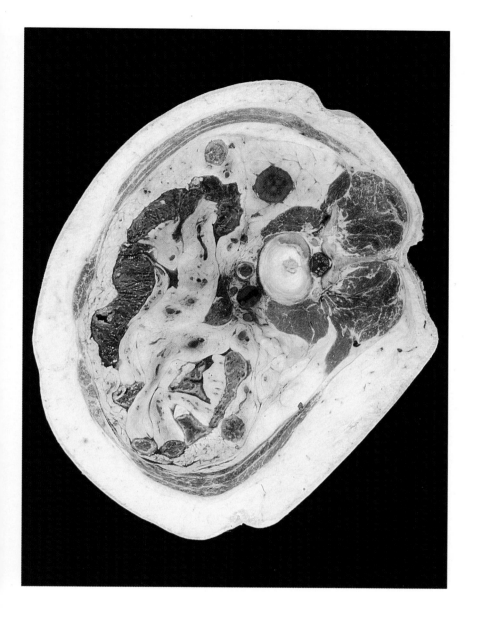

Transverse **Abdomen**

Plate 25

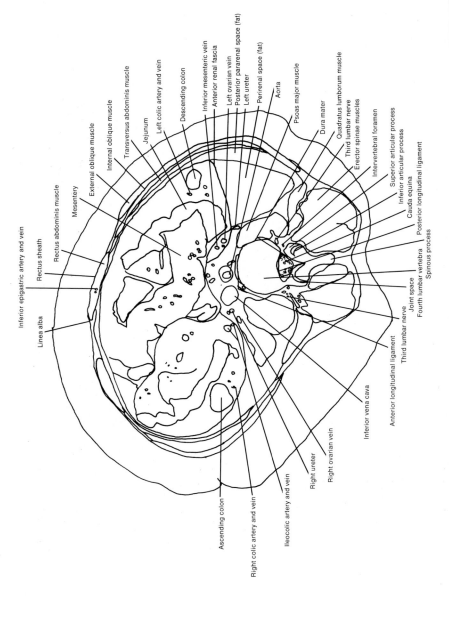

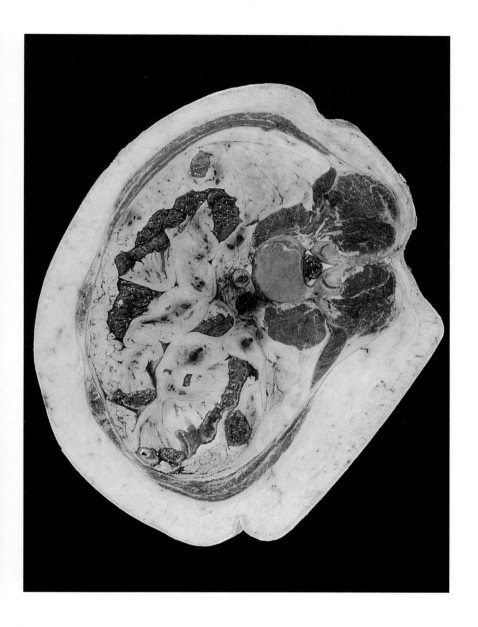

Transverse **Abdomen**

Plate 26

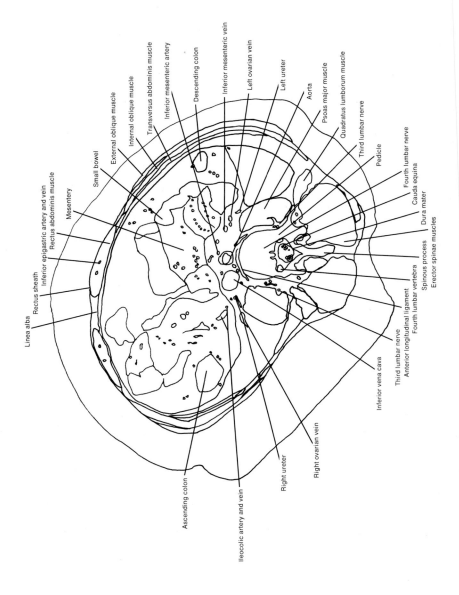

Linea alba
Rectus sheath
Inferior epigastric artery and vein
Rectus abdominis muscle
Mesentery
Small bowel
External oblique muscle
Internal oblique muscle
Transversus abdominis muscle
Inferior mesenteric artery
Descending colon
Inferior mesenteric vein
Left ovarian vein
Left ureter
Aorta
Psoas major muscle
Quadratus lumborum muscle
Third lumbar nerve
Pedicle
Fourth lumbar nerve
Cauda equina
Dura mater
Spinous process
Erector spinae muscles
Fourth lumbar vertebra
Anterior longitudinal ligament
Third lumbar nerve
Inferior vena cava
Right ovarian vein
Right ureter
Ileocolic artery and vein
Ascending colon

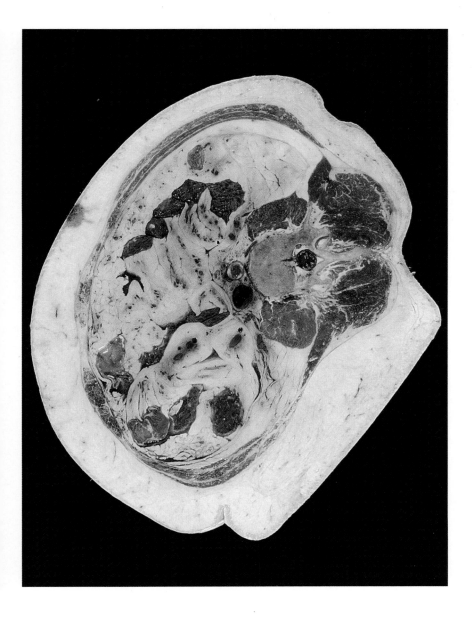

Transverse **Abdomen**

Plate 27

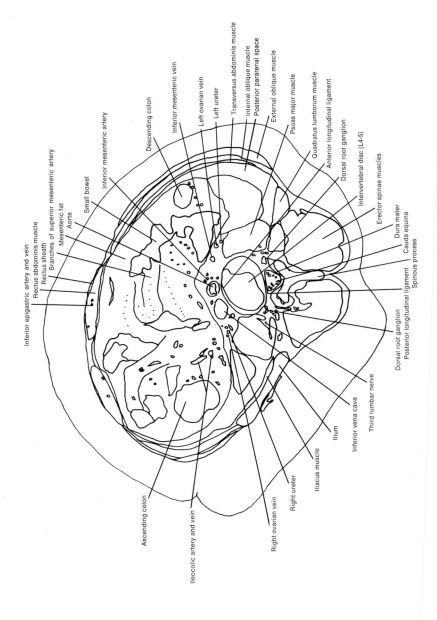

Inferior epigastric artery and vein
Rectus abdominis muscle
Rectus sheath
Branches of superior mesenteric artery
Mesenteric fat
Aorta
Small bowel
Inferior mesenteric artery
Descending colon
Inferior mesenteric vein
Left ovarian vein
Left ureter
Transversus abdominis muscle
Internal oblique muscle
Posterior pararenal space
External oblique muscle
Psoas major muscle
Quadratus lumborum muscle
Anterior longitudinal ligament
Dorsal root ganglion
Intervertebral disc (L4-5)
Erector spinae muscles
Dura mater
Cauda equina
Spinous process
Posterior longitudinal ligament
Dorsal root ganglion
Third lumbar nerve
Inferior vena cava
Ilium
Iliacus muscle
Right ureter
Right ovarian vein
Ileocolic artery and vein
Ascending colon

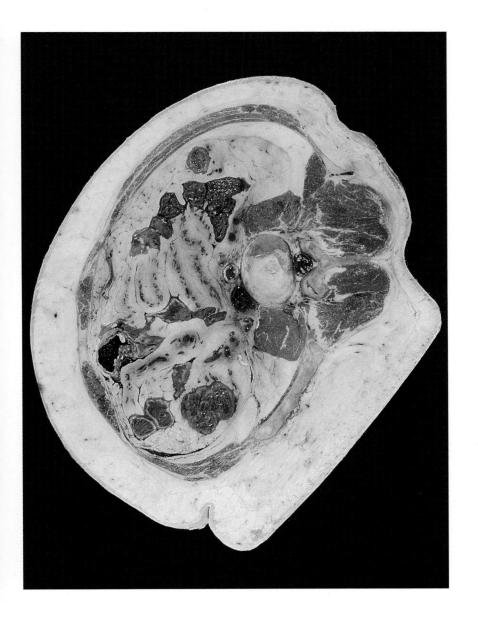

Transverse **Abdomen**

TRANSVERSE   Pelvis—Female   *Plates 28–52*

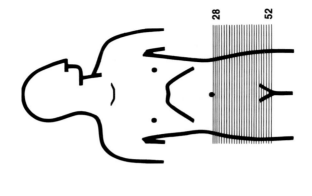

28

52

Female Reproductive System

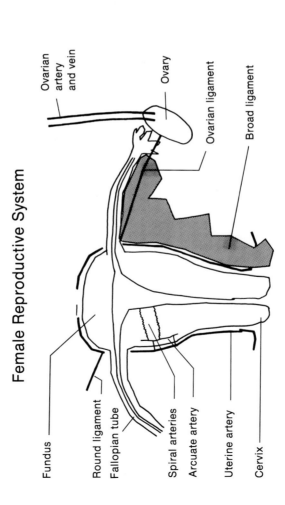

Ovarian
artery
and vein

Ovary

Ovarian ligament

Broad ligament

Fundus

Round ligament

Fallopian tube

Spiral arteries

Arcuate artery

Uterine artery

Cervix

Plate 28

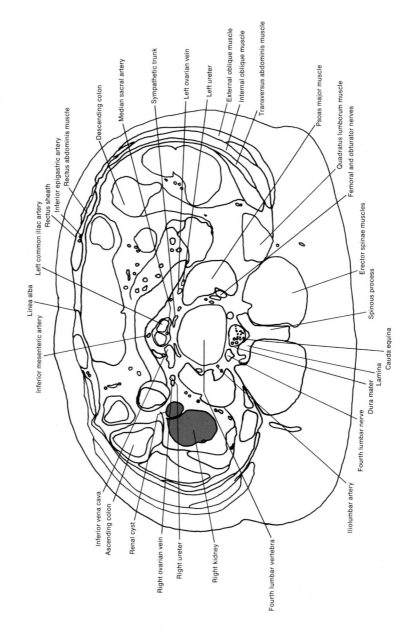

- Linea alba
- Left common iliac artery
- Rectus sheath
- Inferior epigastric artery
- Rectus abdominis muscle
- Descending colon
- Median sacral artery
- Sympathetic trunk
- Left ovarian vein
- Left ureter
- External oblique muscle
- Internal oblique muscle
- Transversus abdominis muscle
- Psoas major muscle
- Quadratus lumborum muscle
- Femoral and obturator nerves
- Erector spinae muscles
- Spinous process
- Cauda equina
- Lamina
- Dura mater
- Fourth lumbar nerve
- Iliolumbar artery
- Fourth lumbar vertebra
- Right kidney
- Right ureter
- Right ovarian vein
- Renal cyst
- Ascending colon
- Inferior vena cava
- Inferior mesenteric artery

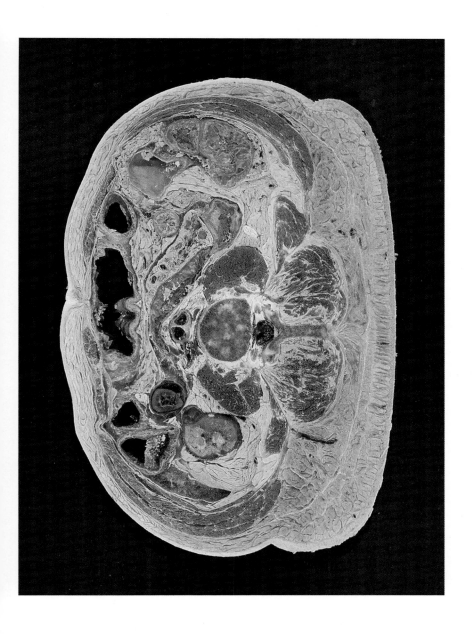

Transverse **Pelvis—Female**

Plate 29

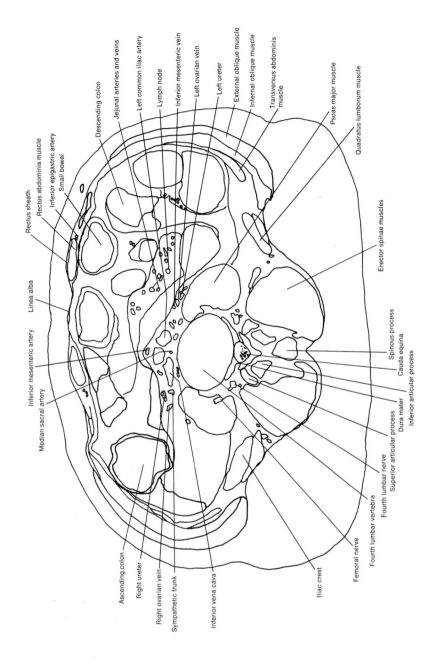

Rectus sheath
Rectus abdominis muscle
Inferior epigastric artery
Small bowel

Linea alba

Inferior mesenteric artery

Median sacral artery

Ascending colon
Right ureter
Right ovarian vein
Sympathetic trunk

Inferior vena cava

Descending colon
Jejunal arteries and veins
Left common iliac artery
Lymph node
Inferior mesenteric vein
Left ovarian vein
Left ureter
External oblique muscle
Internal oblique muscle
Transversus abdominis
muscle

Psoas major muscle
Quadratus lumborum muscle

Erector spinae muscles

Spinous process
Cauda equina
Inferior articular process

Superior articular process
Dura mater
Fourth lumbar nerve
Fourth lumbar vertebra

Iliac crest

Femoral nerve

Transverse **Pelvis—Female**

Plate 30

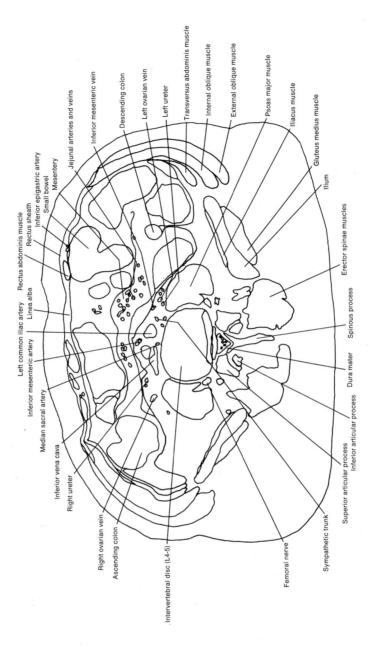

Rectus abdominis muscle
Left common iliac artery
Rectus sheath
Inferior epigastric artery
Small bowel
Mesentery
Linea alba
Inferior mesenteric artery
Jejunal arteries and veins
Inferior mesenteric vein
Descending colon
Left ovarian vein
Left ureter
Transversus abdominis muscle
Internal oblique muscle
External oblique muscle
Psoas major muscle
Iliacus muscle
Gluteus medius muscle
Ilium
Erector spinae muscles
Median sacral artery
Inferior vena cava
Right ureter
Right ovarian vein
Ascending colon
Intervertebral disc (L4-5)
Femoral nerve
Sympathetic trunk
Superior articular process
Inferior articular process
Dura mater
Spinous process

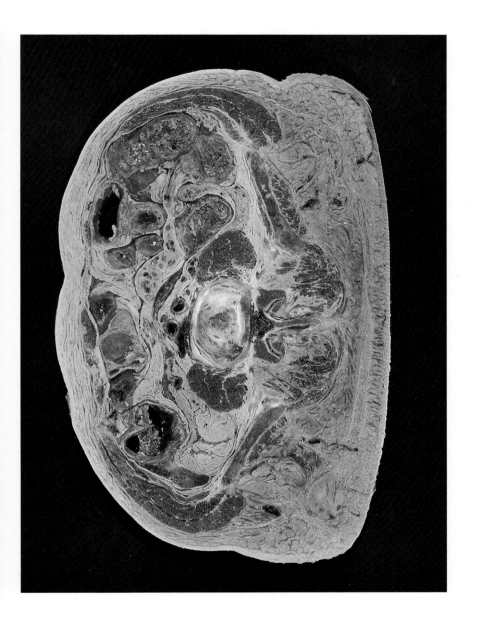

Transverse **Pelvis—Female**

Plate 31

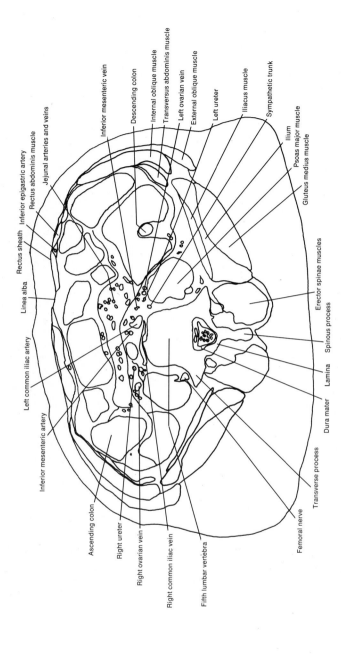

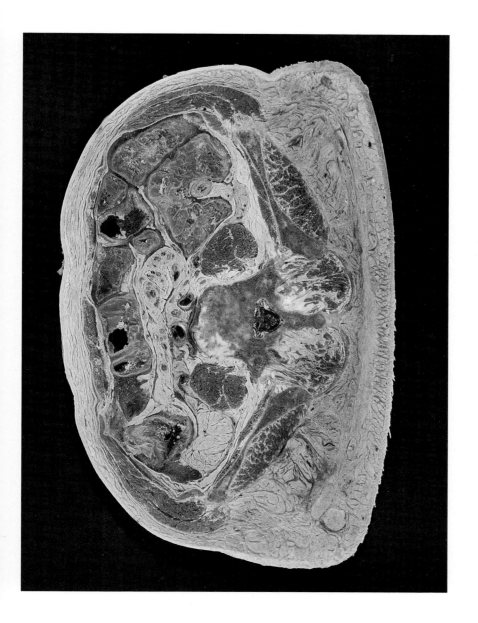

Transverse **Pelvis—Female**

Plate 32

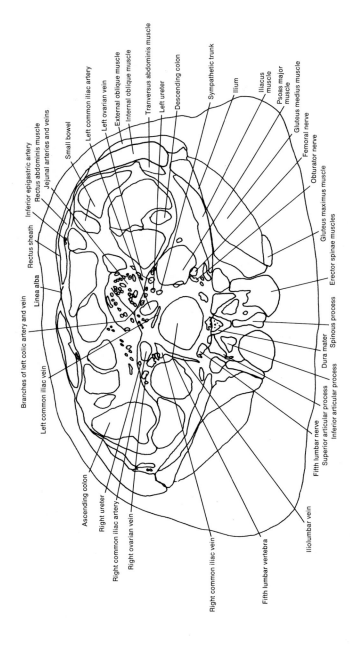

Branches of left colic artery and vein
Inferior epigastric artery
Rectus abdominis muscle
Jejunal arteries and veins
Rectus sheath
Small bowel
Linea alba
Left common iliac artery
Left ovarian vein
External oblique muscle
Internal oblique muscle
Tranversus abdominis muscle
Left ureter
Descending colon
Sympathetic trunk
Ilium
Iliacus muscle
Psoas major muscle
Gluteus medius muscle
Femoral nerve
Obturator nerve
Gluteus maximus muscle
Erector spinae muscles
Spinous process
Dura mater
Inferior articular process
Superior articular process
Fifth lumbar nerve
Left common iliac vein
Ascending colon
Right ureter
Right common iliac artery
Right ovarian vein
Right common iliac vein
Fifth lumbar vertebra
Iliolumbar vein

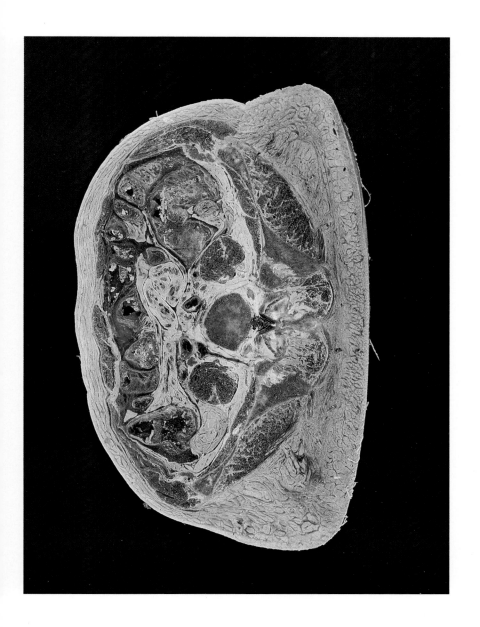

Transverse **Pelvis—Female**

Plate 33

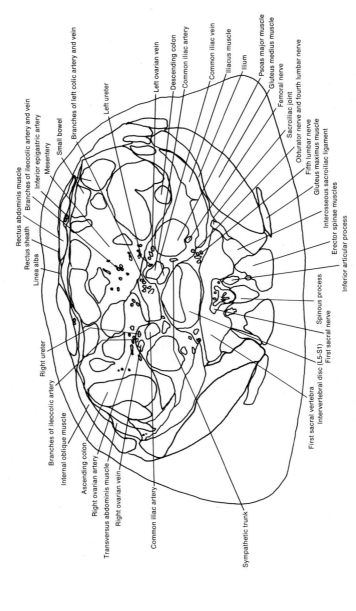

Rectus abdominis muscle
Rectus sheath
Linea alba
Right ureter
Branches of ileocolic artery
Internal oblique muscle
Ascending colon
Right ovarian artery
Transversus abdominis muscle
Right ovarian vein
Common iliac artery
Sympathetic trunk

Branches of ileocolic artery and vein
Inferior epigastric artery
Mesentery
Small bowel
Branches of left colic artery and vein
Left ureter
Left ovarian vein
Descending colon
Common iliac artery
Common iliac vein
Iliacus muscle
Ilium
Psoas major muscle
Gluteus medius muscle
Femoral nerve
Sacroiliac joint
Obturator nerve and fourth lumbar nerve
Fifth lumbar nerve
Gluteus maximus muscle
Interosseous sacroiliac ligament
Erector spinae muscles
Inferior articular process

First sacral vertebra
Intervertebral disc (L5–S1)
First sacral nerve
Spinous process

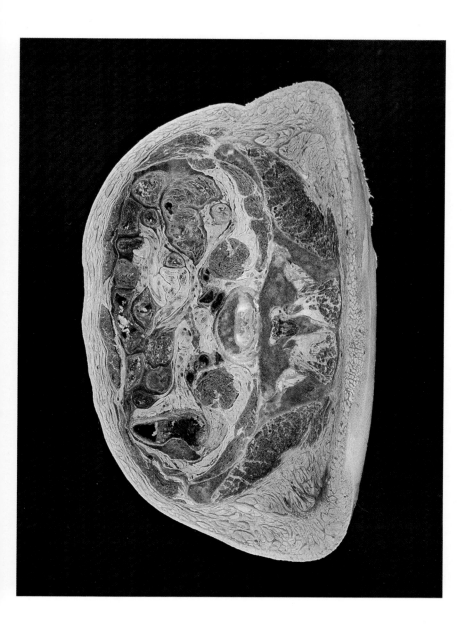

Transverse **Pelvis—Female**

Plate 34

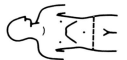

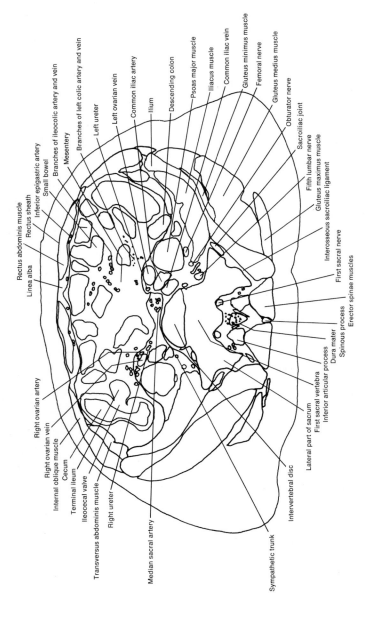

Rectus abdominis muscle
Rectus sheath
Inferior epigastric artery
Small bowel
Branches of ileocolic artery and vein
Mesentery
Branches of left colic artery and vein
Left ureter
Left ovarian vein
Common iliac artery
Ilium
Descending colon
Psoas major muscle
Iliacus muscle
Common iliac vein
Gluteus minimus muscle
Femoral nerve
Gluteus medius muscle
Obturator nerve
Sacroiliac joint
Fifth lumbar nerve
Gluteus maximus muscle
Interosseous sacroiliac ligament
First sacral nerve
Erector spinae muscles
Dura mater
Spinous process
Inferior articular process
First sacral vertebra
Lateral part of sacrum
Intervertebral disc
Sympathetic trunk
Median sacral artery
Right ureter
Transversus abdominis muscle
Ileocecal valve
Terminal ileum
Cecum
Internal oblique muscle
Right ovarian vein
Right ovarian artery
Linea alba

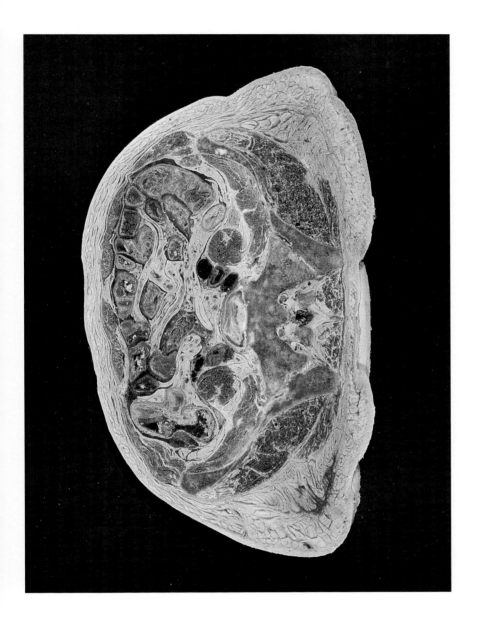

Transverse **Pelvis—Female**

Plate 35

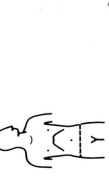

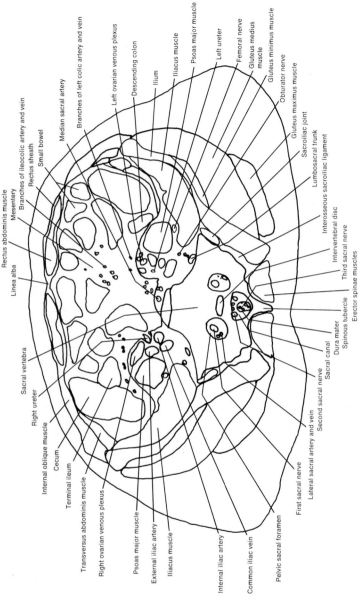

- Rectus abdominis muscle
- Mesentery
- Branches of ileocolic artery and vein
- Rectus sheath
- Small bowel
- Median sacral artery
- Branches of left colic artery and vein
- Left ovarian venous plexus
- Descending colon
- Ilium
- Iliacus muscle
- Psoas major muscle
- Left ureter
- Femoral nerve
- Gluteus medius muscle
- Gluteus minimus muscle
- Obturator nerve
- Gluteus maximus muscle
- Sacroiliac joint
- Lumbosacral trunk
- Interosseous sacroiliac ligament
- Intervertebral disc
- Third sacral nerve
- Erector spinae muscles
- Spinous tubercle
- Dura mater
- Sacral canal
- Second sacral nerve
- Lateral sacral artery and vein
- First sacral nerve
- Pelvic sacral foramen
- Internal iliac artery
- Common iliac vein
- Iliacus muscle
- External iliac artery
- Psoas major muscle
- Right ovarian venous plexus
- Transversus abdominis muscle
- Terminal ileum
- Cecum
- Internal oblique muscle
- Right ureter
- Sacral vertebra
- Linea alba

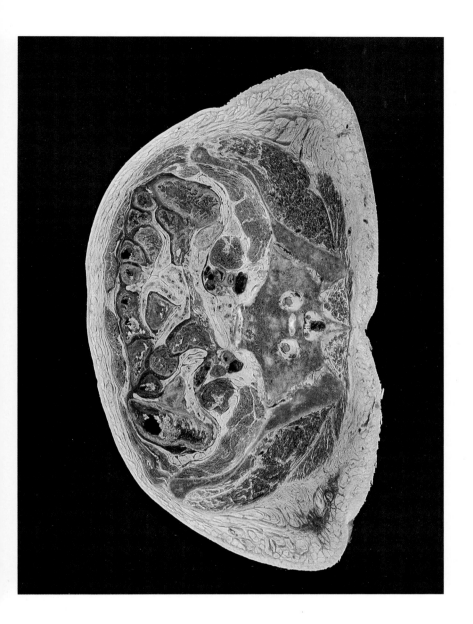

Transverse **Pelvis—Female**

Plate 36

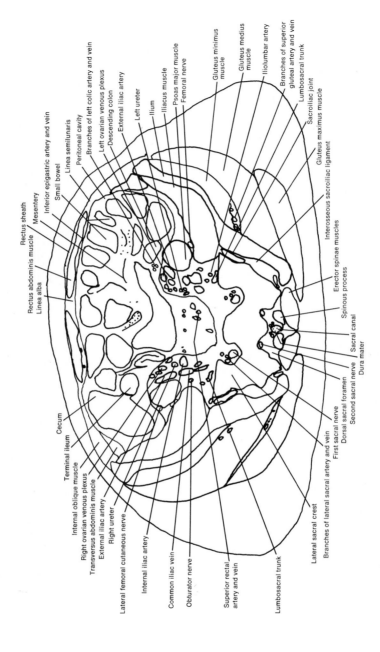

Rectus abdominis muscle
Rectus sheath
Mesentery
Linea alba
Inferior epigastric artery and vein
Small bowel
Cecum
Linea semilunaris
Terminal ileum
Peritoneal cavity
Internal oblique muscle
Branches of left colic artery and vein
Right ovarian venous plexus
Left ovarian venous plexus
Transversus abdominis muscle
Descending colon
External iliac artery
External iliac artery
Right ureter
Left ureter
Lateral femoral cutaneous nerve
Ilium
Iliacus muscle
Internal iliac artery
Psoas major muscle
Common iliac vein
Femoral nerve
Obturator nerve
Gluteus minimus muscle
Gluteus medius muscle
Superior rectal artery and vein
Iliolumbar artery
Branches of superior gluteal artery and vein
Lumbosacral trunk
Lumbosacral trunk
Lateral sacral crest
Sacroiliac joint
Branches of lateral sacral artery and vein
Gluteus maximus muscle
First sacral nerve
Interosseous sacroiliac ligament
Dorsal sacral foramen
Erector spinae muscles
Second sacral nerve
Spinous process
Sacral canal
Dura mater

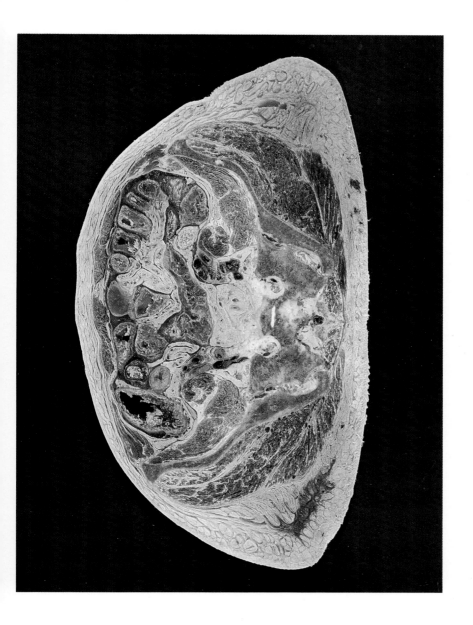

Transverse **Pelvis—Female**

Plate 37

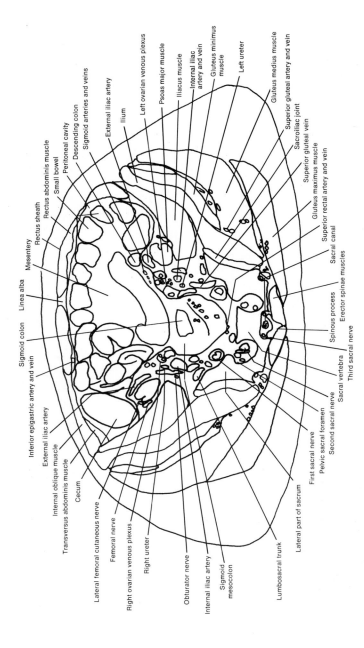

Rectus sheath
Rectus abdominis muscle
Small bowel
Peritoneal cavity
Descending colon
Sigmoid arteries and veins
External iliac artery
Ilium
Left ovarian venous plexus
Psoas major muscle
Iliacus muscle
Internal iliac artery and vein
Gluteus minimus muscle
Left ureter
Gluteus medius muscle
Superior gluteal artery and vein
Sacroiliac joint
Superior gluteal vein
Gluteus maximus muscle
Superior rectal artery and vein
Sacral canal
Erector spinae muscles
Spinous process
Third sacral nerve
Sacral vertebra
Second sacral nerve
Pelvic sacral foramen
First sacral nerve
Lateral part of sacrum
Lumbosacral trunk
Sigmoid mesocolon
Internal iliac artery
Obturator nerve
Right ureter
Right ovarian venous plexus
Femoral nerve
Lateral femoral cutaneous nerve
Transversus abdominis muscle
Cecum
Internal oblique muscle
External iliac artery
Inferior epigastric artery and vein
Sigmoid colon
Linea alba
Mesentery

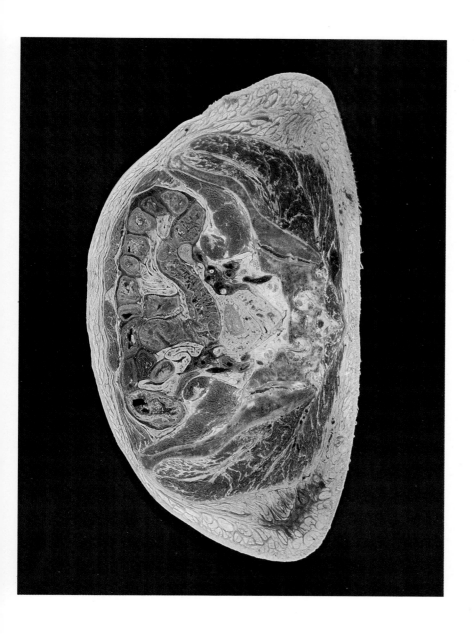

Transverse **Pelvis—Female**

Plate 38

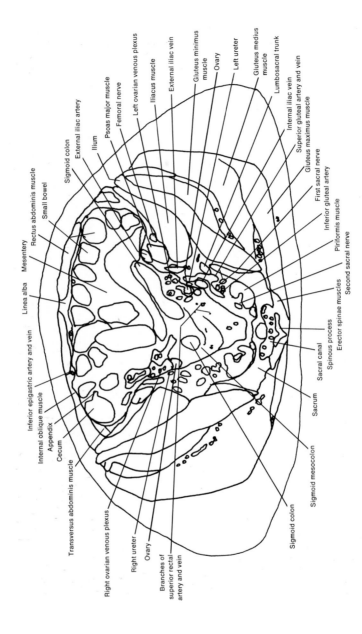

Linea alba
Mesentery
Rectus abdominis muscle
Small bowel
Sigmoid colon
External iliac artery
Ilium
Psoas major muscle
Femoral nerve
Left ovarian venous plexus
Iliacus muscle
External iliac vein
Gluteus minimus muscle
Ovary
Left ureter
Gluteus medius muscle
Lumbosacral trunk
Internal iliac vein
Superior gluteal artery and vein
Gluteus maximus muscle
First sacral nerve
Inferior gluteal artery
Piriformis muscle
Second sacral nerve
Erector spinae muscles
Spinous process
Sacral canal
Sacrum
Sigmoid mesocolon
Sigmoid colon
Branches of superior rectal artery and vein
Ovary
Right ureter
Right ovarian venous plexus
Transversus abdominis muscle
Cecum
Appendix
Internal oblique muscle
Inferior epigastric artery and vein

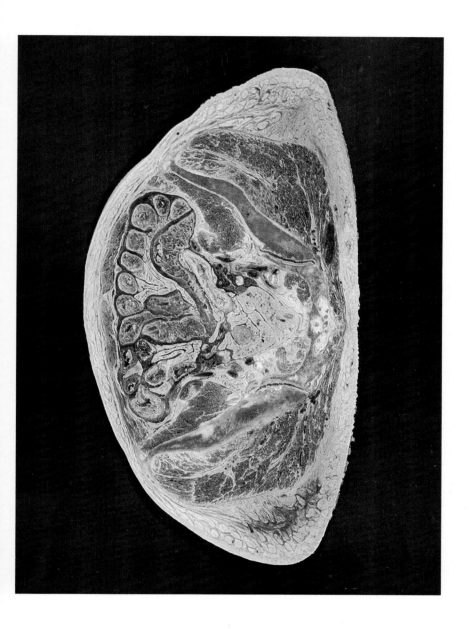

Transverse **Pelvis—Female**

85

Plate 39

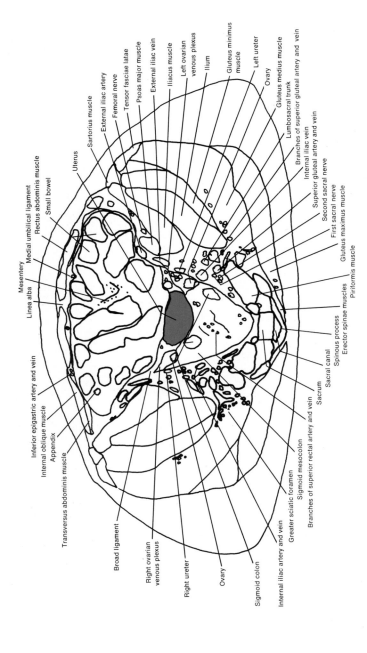

Inferior epigastric artery and vein
Internal oblique muscle
Appendix
Transversus abdominis muscle

Mesentery
Linea alba
Medial umbilical ligament
Rectus abdominis muscle
Small bowel

Uterus
Sartorius muscle
External iliac artery
Femoral nerve
Tensor fasciae latae
Psoas major muscle
External iliac vein
Iliacus muscle
Left ovarian venous plexus
Ilium
Gluteus minimus muscle
Left ureter
Ovary
Gluteus medius muscle
Lumbosacral trunk
Branches of superior gluteal artery and vein
Internal iliac vein
Superior gluteal artery and vein
Second sacral nerve
First sacral nerve
Gluteus maximus muscle
Piriformis muscle

Broad ligament
Right ovarian venous plexus
Right ureter
Ovary
Sigmoid colon
Internal iliac artery and vein
Greater sciatic foramen
Sigmoid mesocolon
Branches of superior rectal artery and vein

Sacrum
Sacral canal
Spinous process
Erector spinae muscles

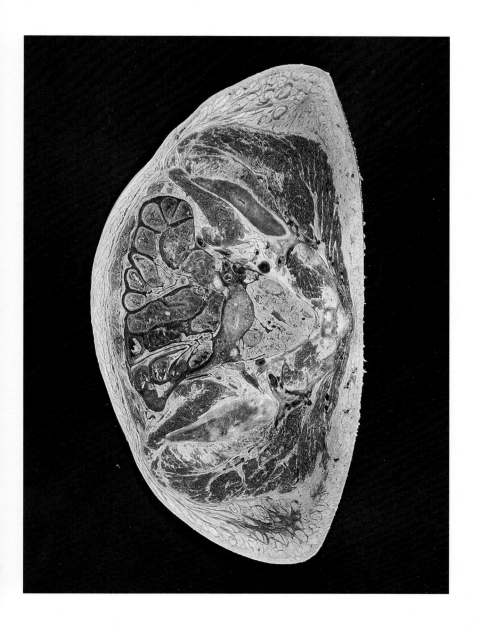

Transverse **Pelvis—Female**

Plate 40

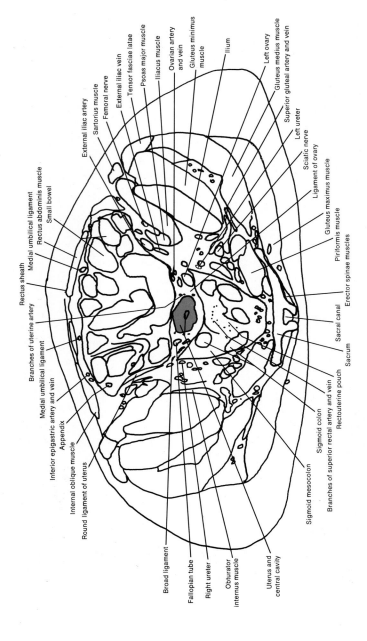

Rectus sheath
Medial umbilical ligament
Rectus abdominis muscle
Small bowel

External iliac artery
Sartorius muscle
Femoral nerve
External iliac vein
Tensor fasciae latae
Psoas major muscle
Iliacus muscle
Ovarian artery and vein
Gluteus minimus muscle
Ilium
Left ovary
Gluteus medius muscle
Superior gluteal artery and vein
Left ureter
Sciatic nerve
Ligament of ovary
Gluteus maximus muscle
Piriformis muscle
Erector spinae muscles
Sacral canal
Sacrum
Rectouterine pouch
Branches of superior rectal artery and vein
Sigmoid colon
Sigmoid mesocolon

Branches of uterine artery
Medial umbilical ligament
Inferior epigastric artery and vein
Appendix
Internal oblique muscle
Round ligament of uterus

Broad ligament
Fallopian tube
Right ureter
Obturator internus muscle
Uterus and central cavity

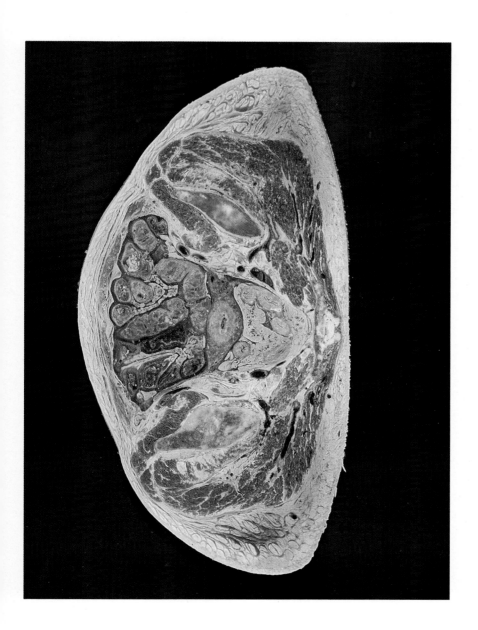

Transverse **Pelvis—Female**

Plate 41

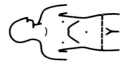

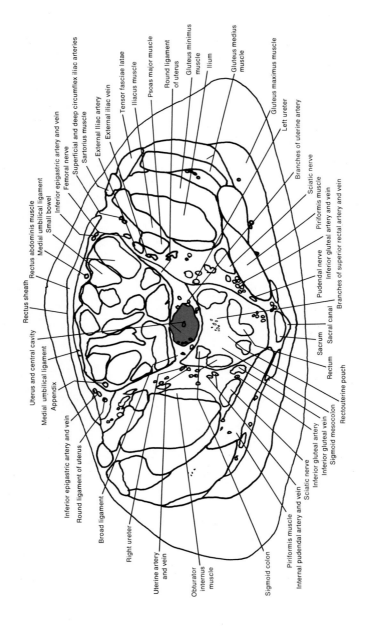

- Uterus and central cavity
- Medial umbilical ligament
- Appendix
- Rectus sheath
- Rectus abdominis muscle
- Medial umbilical ligament
- Small bowel
- Inferior epigastric artery and vein
- Femoral nerve
- Superficial and deep circumflex iliac arteries
- Sartorius muscle
- External iliac artery
- External iliac vein
- Tensor fasciae latae
- Iliacus muscle
- Psoas major muscle
- Round ligament of uterus
- Gluteus minimus muscle
- Ilium
- Gluteus medius muscle
- Gluteus maximus muscle
- Branches of uterine artery
- Left ureter
- Sciatic nerve
- Piriformis muscle
- Inferior gluteal artery and vein
- Branches of superior rectal artery and vein
- Pudendal nerve
- Sacral canal
- Sacrum
- Rectum
- Rectouterine pouch
- Sigmoid mesocolon
- Inferior gluteal vein
- Inferior gluteal artery
- Sciatic nerve
- Internal pudendal artery and vein
- Piriformis muscle
- Sigmoid colon
- Obturator internus muscle
- Uterine artery and vein
- Right ureter
- Broad ligament
- Round ligament of uterus
- Inferior epigastric artery and vein

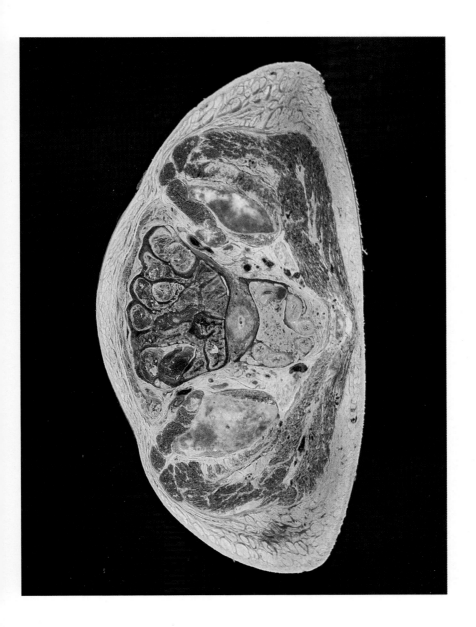

Transverse **Pelvis—Female**

Plate 42

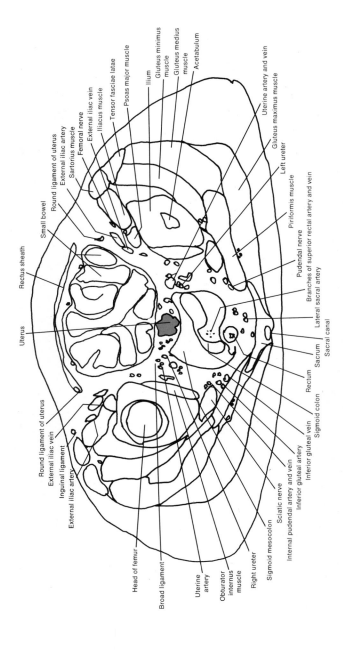

Small bowel

Rectus sheath

Uterus

Round ligament of uterus
External iliac artery
Sartorius muscle
Femoral nerve
External iliac vein
Iliacus muscle
Tensor fasciae latae
Psoas major muscle
Ilium
Gluteus minimus muscle
Gluteus medius muscle
Acetabulum
Uterine artery and vein
Gluteus maximus muscle
Left ureter
Piriformis muscle
Pudendal nerve
Branches of superior rectal artery and vein
Lateral sacral artery
Sacral canal
Sacrum
Rectum
Sigmoid colon
Inferior gluteal vein
Inferior gluteal artery
Internal pudendal artery and vein
Sciatic nerve
Sigmoid mesocolon
Right ureter
Obturator internus muscle
Uterine artery
Broad ligament
Head of femur
External iliac artery
Inguinal ligament
External iliac vein
Round ligament of uterus
Round ligament of uterus

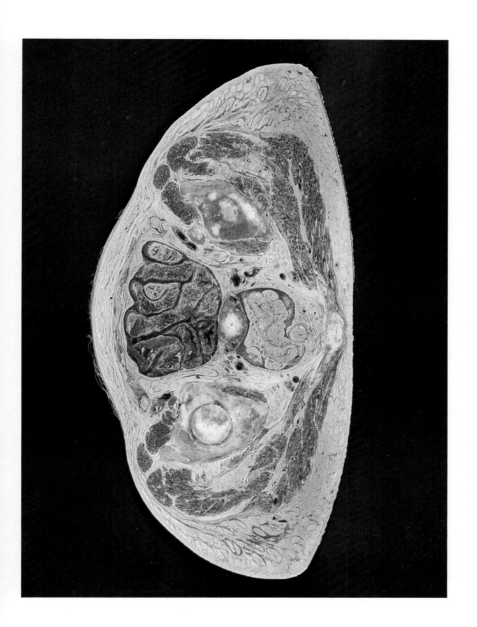

Transverse **Pelvis—Female**

Plate 43

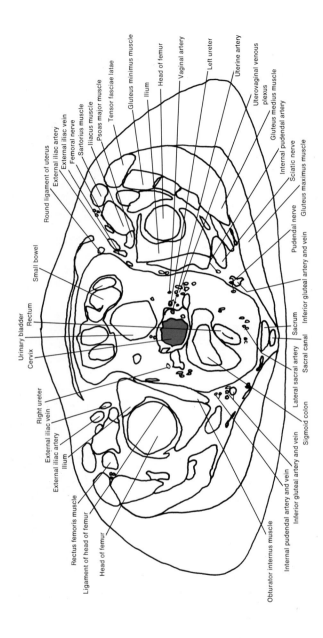

Round ligament of uterus
External iliac artery
External iliac vein
Femoral nerve
Sartorius muscle
Iliacus muscle
Psoas major muscle
Tensor fasciae latae
Gluteus minimus muscle
Ilium
Head of femur
Vaginal artery
Left ureter
Uterine artery
Uterovaginal venous plexus
Gluteus medius muscle
Internal pudendal artery
Sciatic nerve
Gluteus maximus muscle
Pudendal nerve
Inferior gluteal artery and vein
Sacrum
Sacral canal
Lateral sacral artery
Sigmoid colon
Inferior gluteal artery and vein
Internal pudendal artery and vein
Obturator internus muscle
Head of femur
Ligament of head of femur
Rectus femoris muscle
Ilium
External iliac artery
External iliac vein
Right ureter
Urinary bladder
Cervix
Rectum
Small bowel

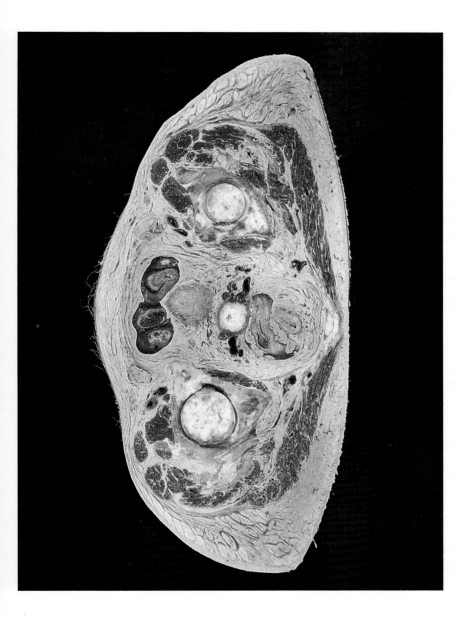

Transverse **Pelvis—Female**

Plate 44

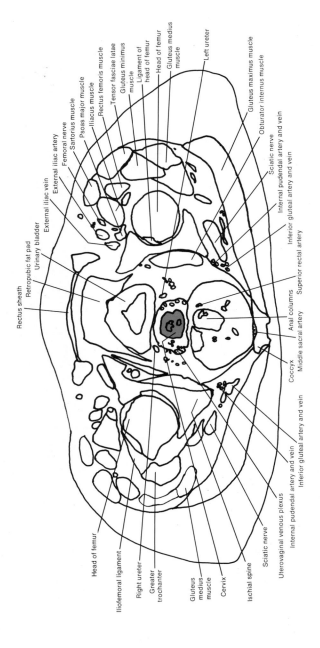

Rectus sheath
Retropubic fat pad
Urinary bladder
External iliac vein
External iliac artery
Femoral nerve
Sartorius muscle
Psoas major muscle
Iliacus muscle
Rectus femoris muscle
Tensor fasciae latae
Gluteus minimus muscle
Ligament of head of femur
Head of femur
Gluteus medius muscle
Left ureter
Gluteus maximus muscle
Obturator internus muscle
Sciatic nerve
Internal pudendal artery and vein
Inferior gluteal artery and vein
Superior rectal artery
Middle sacral artery
Coccyx
Anal columns

Head of femur
Iliofemoral ligament
Right ureter
Greater trochanter
Gluteus medius muscle
Cervix
Ischial spine
Uterovaginal venous plexus
Internal pudendal artery and vein
Inferior gluteal artery and vein
Sciatic nerve

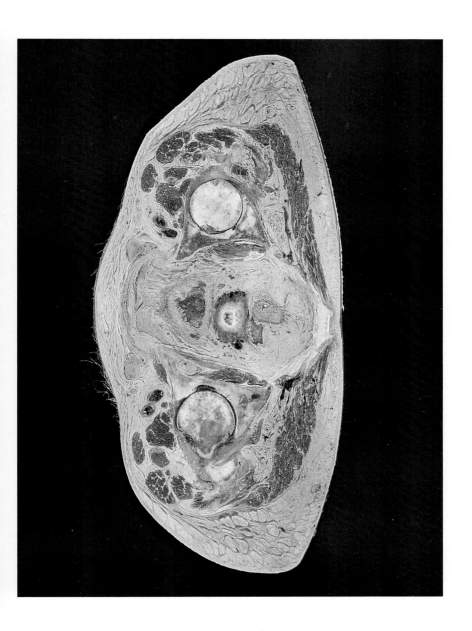

Transverse **Pelvis—Female**

Plate 45

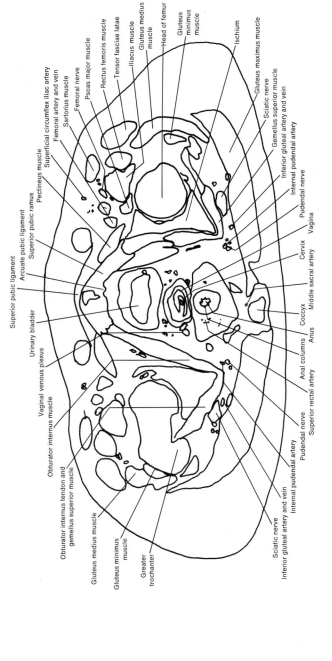

Superior pubic ligament
Arcuate pubic ligament
Superior pubic ramus
Pectineus muscle
Superficial circumflex iliac artery
Femoral artery and vein
Sartorius muscle
Femoral nerve
Rectus femoris muscle
Psoas major muscle
Tensor fasciae latae
Iliacus muscle
Gluteus medius muscle
Head of femur
Gluteus minimus muscle
Ischium
Gluteus maximus muscle
Sciatic nerve
Gemellus superior muscle
Inferior gluteal artery and vein
Internal pudendal artery
Pudendal nerve
Vagina
Cervix
Middle sacral artery
Coccyx
Anus
Anal columns
Superior rectal artery
Pudendal nerve
Internal pudendal artery
Sciatic nerve
Inferior gluteal artery and vein
Greater trochanter
Gluteus minimus muscle
Gluteus medius muscle
Obturator internus tendon and gemellus superior muscle
Obturator internus muscle
Vaginal venous plexus
Urinary bladder
Superior pubic ligament

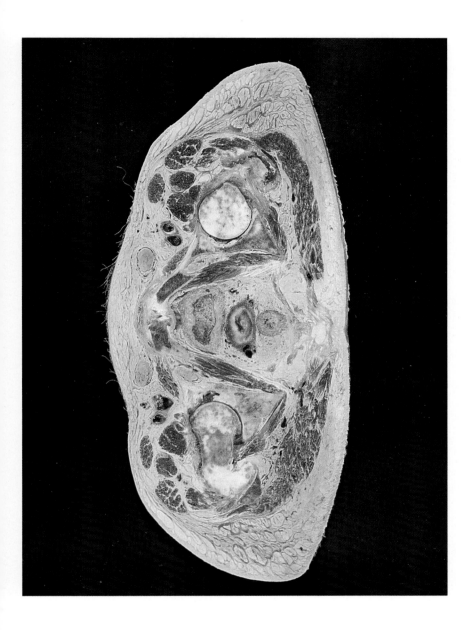

Transverse **Pelvis—Female**

Plate 46

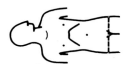

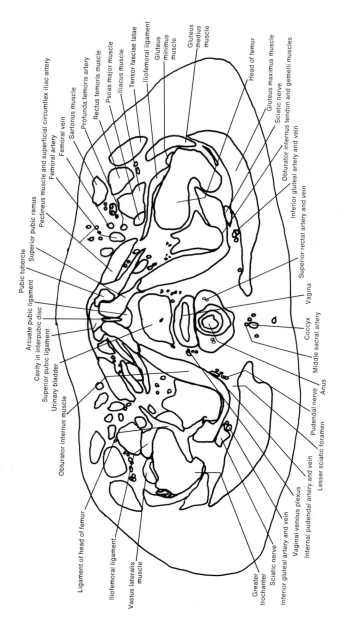

Pubic tubercle
Superior pubic ramus
Pectineus muscle and superficial circumflex iliac artery
Femoral artery
Femoral vein
Sartorius muscle
Profunda femoris artery
Rectus femoris muscle
Psoas major muscle
Iliacus muscle
Tensor fasciae latae
Iliofemoral ligament
Gluteus minimus muscle
Gluteus medius muscle
Head of femur
Gluteus maximus muscle
Sciatic nerve
Obturator internus tendon and vein
Inferior gluteal artery and vein

Arcuate pubic ligament
Cavity in interpubic disc
Superior pubic ligament
Urinary bladder
Obturator internus muscle

Superior rectal artery
Vagina
Coccyx
Middle sacral artery
Anus
Pudendal nerve
Lesser sciatic foramen

Ligament of head of femur
Iliofemoral ligament
Vastus lateralis muscle
Greater trochanter
Sciatic nerve
Inferior gluteal artery and vein
Vaginal venous plexus
Internal pudendal artery and vein

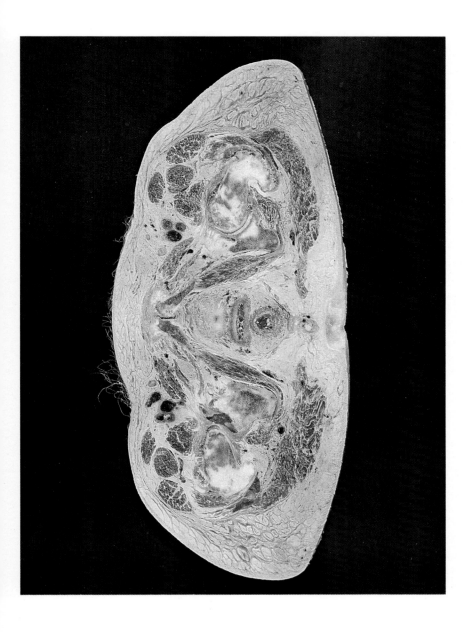

Transverse **Pelvis—Female**

Plate 47

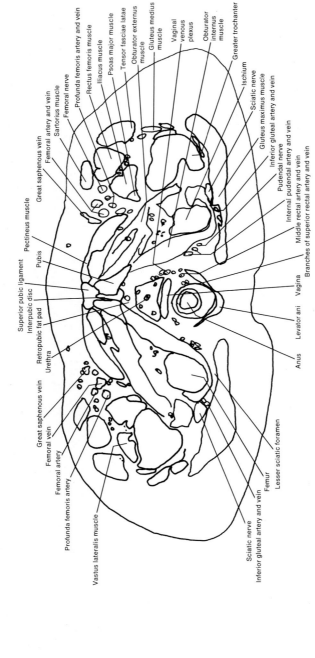

Superior pubic ligament
Interpubic disc
Retropubic fat pad
Urethra

Great saphenous vein
Femoral vein
Femoral artery
Profunda femoris artery

Vastus lateralis muscle

Sciatic nerve
Inferior gluteal artery and vein
Femur
Lesser sciatic foramen

Pectineus muscle
Pubis

Great saphenous vein
Femoral artery and vein
Sartorius muscle
Femoral nerve
Profunda femoris artery and vein
Rectus femoris muscle
Iliacus muscle
Psoas major muscle
Tensor fasciae latae
Obturator externus muscle
Gluteus medius muscle

Vaginal venous plexus
Obturator internus muscle
Greater trochanter

Ischium
Sciatic nerve
Gluteus maximus muscle
Inferior gluteal artery and vein
Pudendal nerve
Internal pudendal artery and vein
Middle rectal artery and vein
Branches of superior rectal artery and vein

Anus
Levator ani
Vagina

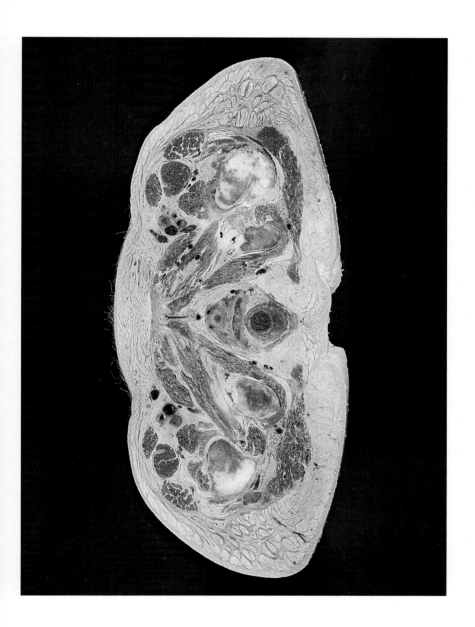

Transverse **Pelvis—Female**

Plate 48

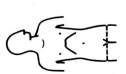

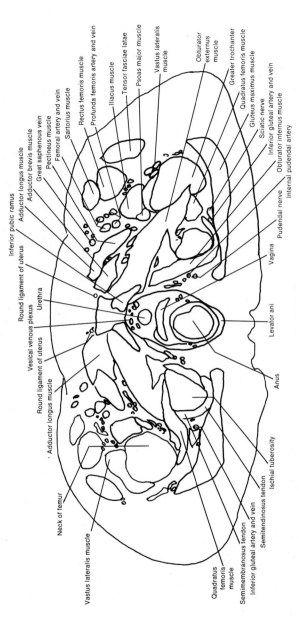

Inferior pubic ramus
Adductor longus muscle
Adductor brevis muscle
Great saphenous vein
Pectineus muscle
Femoral artery and vein
Sartorius muscle
Rectus femoris muscle
Profunda femoris artery and vein
Iliacus muscle
Tensor fasciae latae
Psoas major muscle
Vastus lateralis muscle

Obturator externus muscle
Greater trochanter
Quadratus femoris muscle
Gluteus maximus muscle
Inferior gluteal artery and vein
Sciatic nerve
Obturator internus muscle
Internal pudendal artery
Pudendal nerve

Round ligament of uterus
Urethra
Vesical venous plexus
Round ligament of uterus
Adductor longus muscle

Vagina
Levator ani
Anus

Neck of femur

Vastus lateralis muscle

Quadratus femoris muscle
Semimembranosus tendon
Inferior gluteal artery and vein
Semitendinosus tendon
Ischial tuberosity

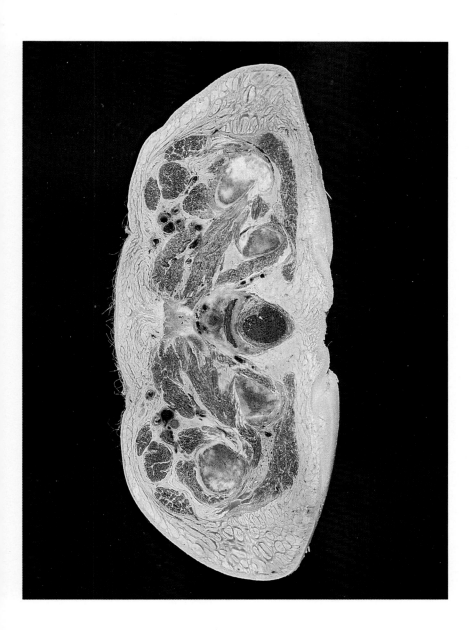

Plate 49

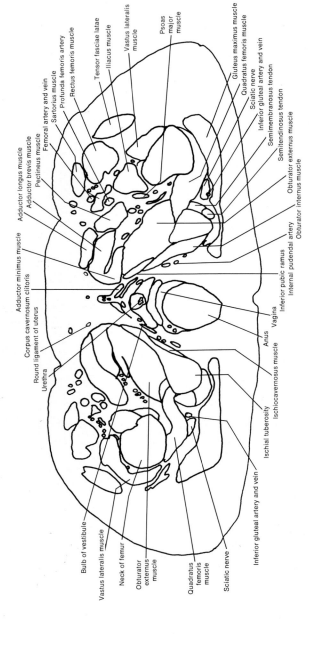

Adductor longus muscle
Adductor brevis muscle
Pectineus muscle
Femoral artery and vein
Sartorius muscle
Profunda femoris artery
Rectus femoris muscle
Tensor fasciae latae
Iliacus muscle
Vastus lateralis muscle
Psoas major muscle
Gluteus maximus muscle
Quadratus femoris muscle
Sciatic nerve
Inferior gluteal artery and vein
Semimembranosus tendon
Semitendinosus tendon
Obturator externus muscle
Obturator internus muscle

Adductor minimus muscle
Corpus cavernosum clitoris
Round ligament of uterus
Urethra

Inferior pubic ramus
Internal pudendal artery
Vagina
Anus
Ischiocavernosus muscle
Ischial tuberosity

Bulb of vestibule
Vastus lateralis muscle
Neck of femur
Obturator externus muscle
Quadratus femoris muscle
Sciatic nerve
Inferior gluteal artery and vein

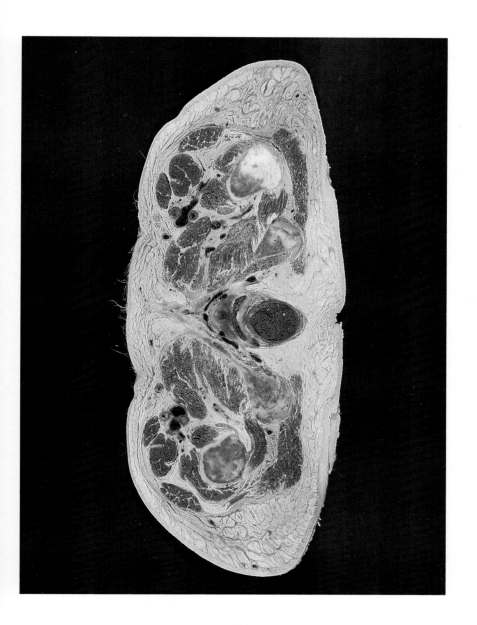

Plate 50

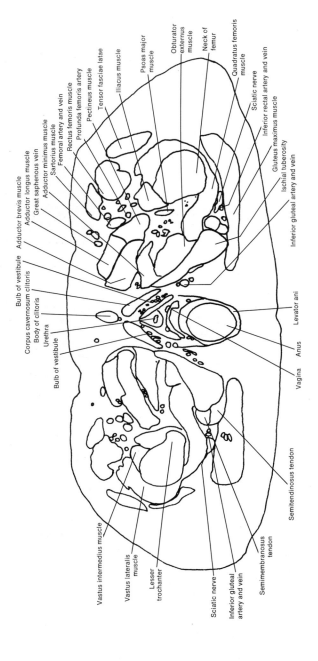

Bulb of vestibule
Adductor brevis muscle
Adductor longus muscle
Great saphenous vein
Adductor minimus muscle
Sartorius muscle
Femoral artery and vein
Rectus femoris muscle
Profunda femoris artery
Pectineus muscle
Tensor fasciae latae
Iliacus muscle
Psoas major muscle
Obturator externus muscle
Neck of femur
Quadratus femoris muscle
Sciatic nerve
Inferior rectal artery and vein
Gluteus maximus muscle
Ischial tuberosity
Inferior gluteal artery and vein

Corpus cavernosum clitoris
Body of clitoris
Urethra
Bulb of vestibule

Levator ani
Anus
Vagina

Vastus intermedius muscle
Vastus lateralis muscle
Lesser trochanter
Sciatic nerve
Inferior gluteal artery and vein
Semimembranosus tendon
Semitendinosus tendon

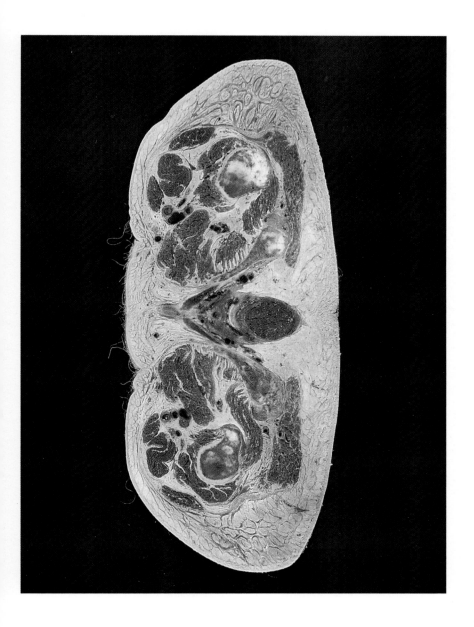

Transverse **Pelvis—Female**

Plate 51

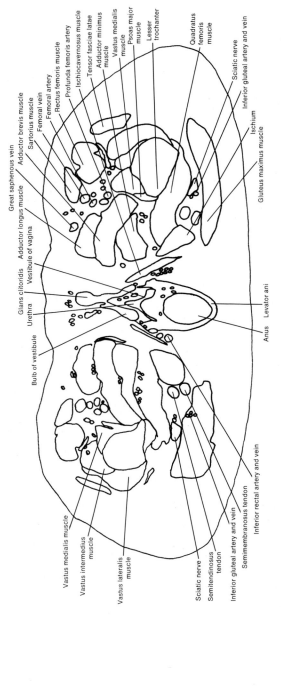

Great saphenous vein

Adductor brevis muscle

Sartorius muscle

Femoral vein

Femoral artery

Rectus femoris muscle

Profunda femoris artery

Ischiocavernosus muscle

Tensor fasciae latae

Adductor minimus muscle

Vastus medialis muscle

Psoas major muscle

Lesser trochanter

Quadratus femoris muscle

Sciatic nerve

Inferior gluteal artery and vein

Ischium

Gluteus maximus muscle

Adductor longus muscle

Vestibule of vagina

Glans clitoridis

Urethra

Bulb of vestibule

Levator ani

Anus

Vastus medialis muscle

Vastus intermedius muscle

Vastus lateralis muscle

Sciatic nerve

Semitendinosus tendon

Inferior gluteal artery and vein

Semimembranosus tendon

Inferior rectal artery and vein

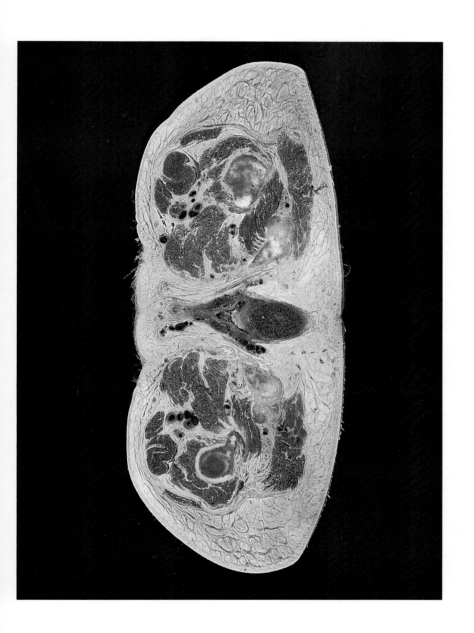

Transverse **Pelvis—Female**

Plate 52

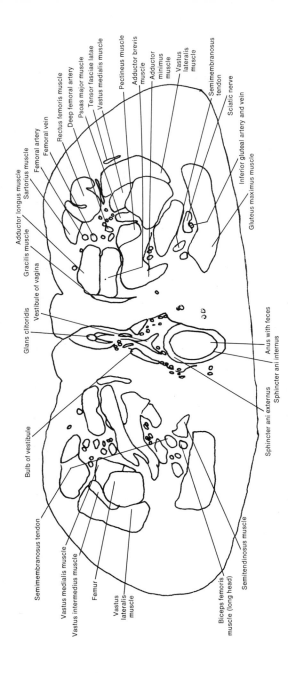

Adductor longus muscle
Sartorius muscle
Gracilis muscle
Vestibule of vagina
Femoral vein
Femoral artery
Rectus femoris muscle
Deep femoral artery
Psoas major muscle
Tensor fasciae latae
Vastus medialis muscle
Pectineus muscle
Adductor brevis muscle
Adductor minimus muscle
Vastus lateralis muscle
Semimembranosus tendon
Sciatic nerve
Inferior gluteal artery and vein
Gluteus maximus muscle

Glans clitoridis
Bulb of vestibule

Anus with feces
Sphincter ani internus
Sphincter ani externus

Semimembranosus tendon
Vastus medialis muscle
Vastus intermedius muscle
Femur
Vastus lateralis muscle
Biceps femoris muscle (long head)
Semitendinosus muscle

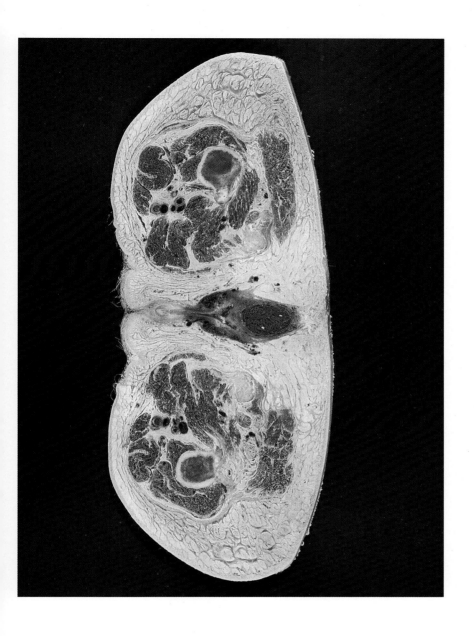

Transverse **Pelvis—Female**

TRANSVERSE   Pelvis—Male   *Plates 53–64*

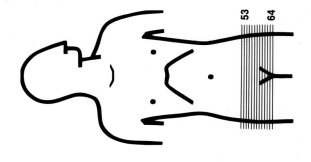

53
64

Plate 53

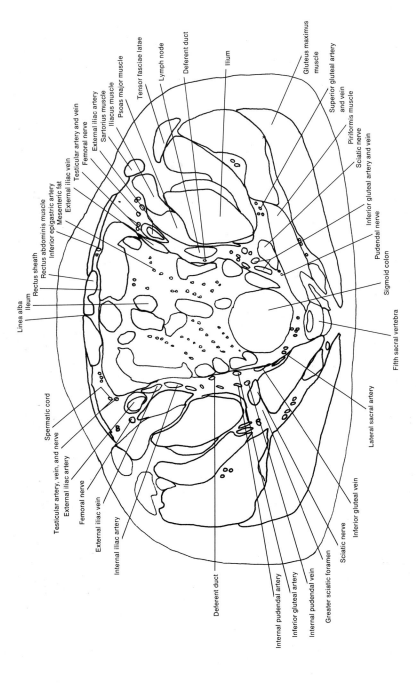

Linea alba
Ileum
Rectus sheath
Rectus abdominis muscle
Inferior epigastric artery
Mesenteric fat
Testicular artery and vein
External iliac vein
External iliac artery
Sartorius muscle
Femoral nerve
Iliacus muscle
Psoas major muscle
Tensor fasciae latae
Lymph node
Deferent duct
Ilium
Gluteus maximus muscle
Superior gluteal artery
Superior gluteal artery and vein
Piriformis muscle
Sciatic nerve
Inferior gluteal artery and vein
Pudendal nerve
Sigmoid colon
Fifth sacral vertebra
Lateral sacral artery
Spermatic cord
Testicular artery, vein, and nerve
External iliac artery
Femoral nerve
External iliac vein
Internal iliac artery
Internal iliac vein
Deferent duct
Internal pudendal artery
Inferior gluteal artery
Internal pudendal vein
Greater sciatic foramen
Sciatic nerve
Inferior gluteal vein

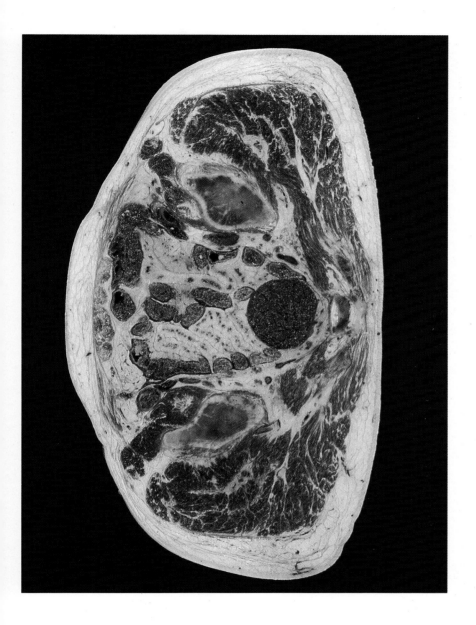

Plate 54

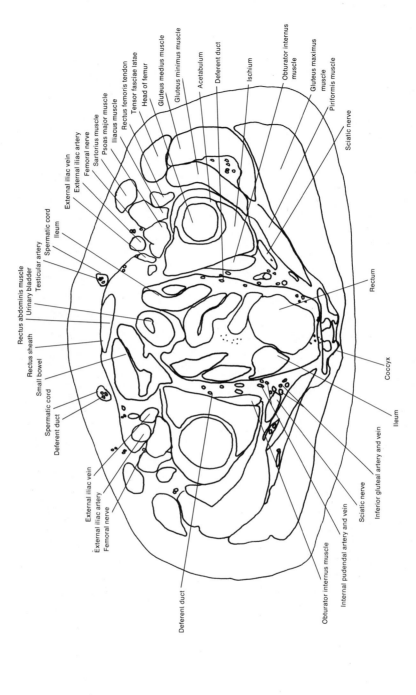

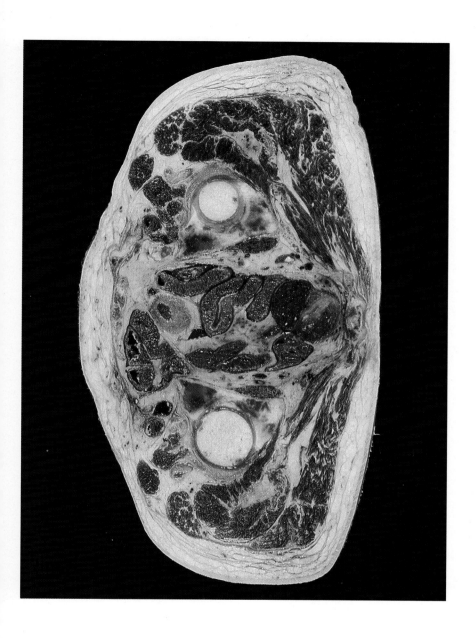

Transverse **Pelvis—Male**

Plate 55

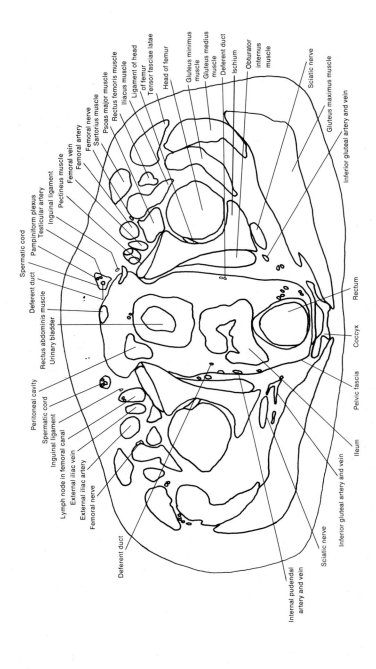

Spermatic cord
Pampiniform plexus
Testicular artery
Inguinal ligament
Pectineus muscle
Femoral vein
Femoral artery
Femoral nerve
Sartorius muscle
Psoas major muscle
Rectus femoris muscle
Iliacus muscle
Ligament of head of femur
Tensor fasciae latae
Head of femur
Gluteus minimus muscle
Gluteus medius muscle
Deferent duct
Ischium
Obturator internus muscle
Sciatic nerve

Deferent duct
Rectus abdominis muscle
Urinary bladder

Gluteus maximus muscle
Inferior gluteal artery and vein

Peritoneal cavity
Spermatic cord
Inguinal ligament
Lymph node in femoral canal
External iliac vein
External iliac artery
Femoral nerve

Deferent duct

Sciatic nerve
Inferior gluteal artery and vein
Internal pudendal artery and vein

Ileum
Pelvic fascia
Coccyx
Rectum

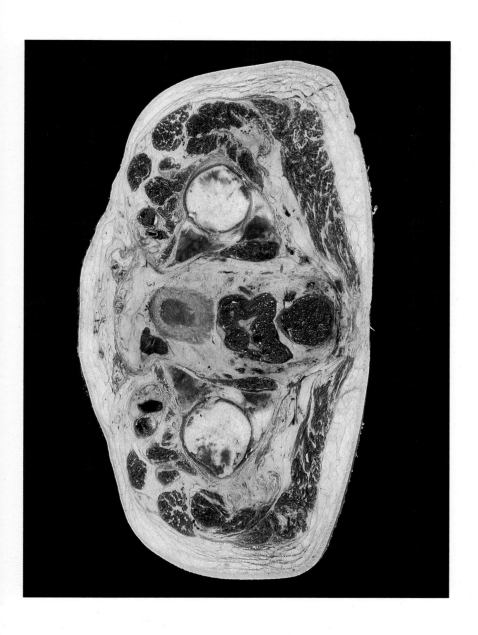

Plate 56

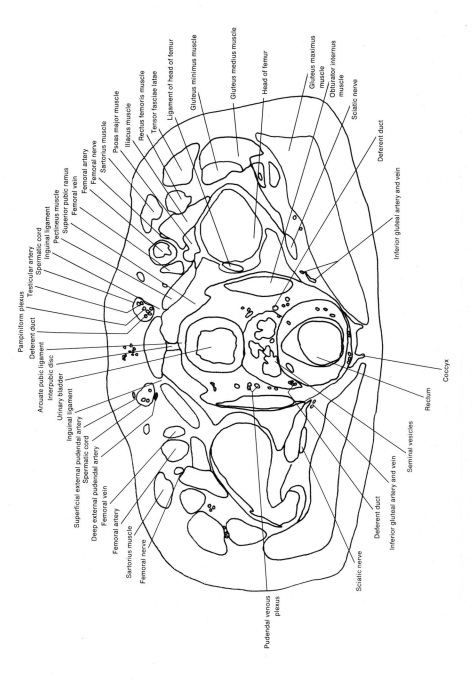

Pampiniform plexus
Deferent duct
Arcuate pubic ligament
Interpubic disc
Urinary bladder
Inguinal ligament
Superficial external pudendal artery
Spermatic cord
Deep external pudendal artery
Femoral vein
Femoral artery
Sartorius muscle
Femoral nerve

Testicular artery
Spermatic cord
Inguinal ligament
Pectineus muscle
Superior pubic ramus
Femoral vein
Femoral artery
Femoral nerve
Sartorius muscle
Psoas major muscle
Iliacus muscle
Rectus femoris muscle
Tensor fasciae latae
Ligament of head of femur
Gluteus minimus muscle
Gluteus medius muscle
Head of femur
Gluteus maximus muscle
Obturator internus muscle
Sciatic nerve

Deferent duct

Inferior gluteal artery and vein

Coccyx

Rectum

Seminal vesicles

Inferior gluteal artery and vein

Deferent duct

Sciatic nerve

Pudendal venous plexus

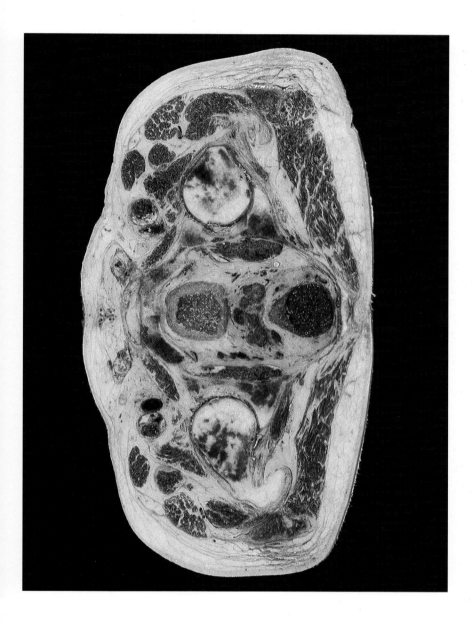

Transverse **Pelvis—Male**

Plate 57

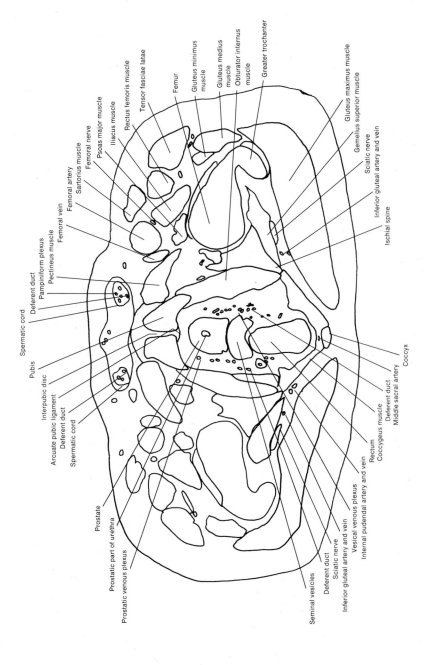

Spermatic cord
Pubis
Interpubic disc
Arcuate pubic ligament
Deferent duct
Spermatic cord
Prostate
Prostatic part of urethra
Prostatic venous plexus

Deferent duct
Pampiniform plexus
Pectineus muscle
Femoral vein
Femoral artery
Sartorius muscle
Femoral nerve
Psoas major muscle
Iliacus muscle
Rectus femoris muscle
Tensor fasciae latae
Femur
Gluteus minimus muscle
Gluteus medius muscle
Obturator internus muscle
Greater trochanter

Gluteus maximus muscle
Gemellus superior muscle
Sciatic nerve
Inferior gluteal artery and vein
Ischial spine
Coccyx
Middle sacral artery
Deferent duct
Rectum
Coccygeus muscle
Internal pudendal artery and vein
Vesical venous plexus
Inferior gluteal artery and vein
Sciatic nerve
Deferent duct
Seminal vesicles

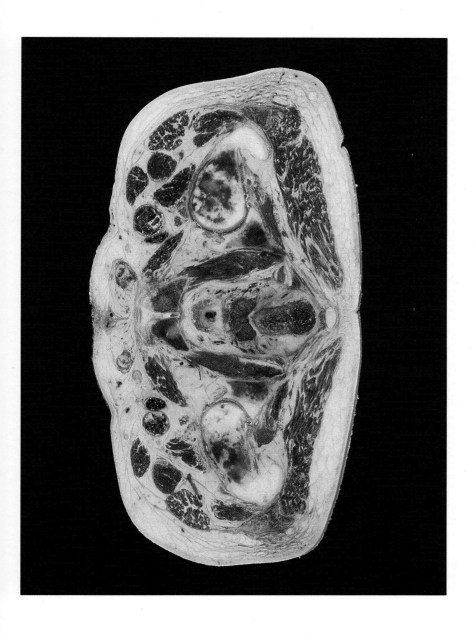

Transverse **Pelvis—Male**

Plate 58

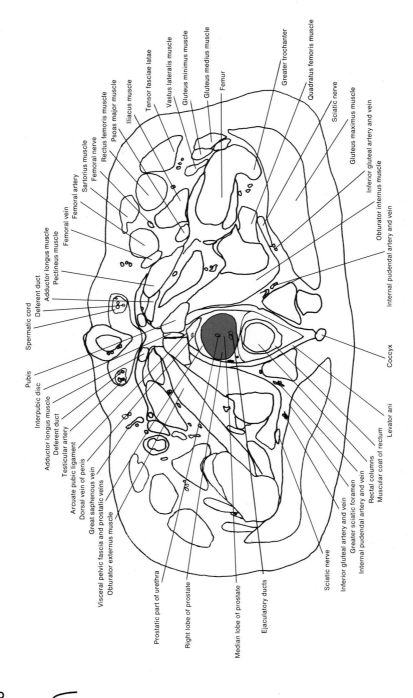

Pubis
Spermatic cord
Deferent duct
Adductor longus muscle
Pectineus muscle
Femoral vein
Femoral artery
Sartorius muscle
Femoral nerve
Rectus femoris muscle
Psoas major muscle
Iliacus muscle
Tensor fasciae latae
Vastus lateralis muscle
Gluteus minimus muscle
Gluteus medius muscle
Femur
Greater trochanter
Quadratus femoris muscle
Sciatic nerve
Gluteus maximus muscle
Inferior gluteal artery and vein
Obturator internus muscle
Internal pudendal artery and vein

Interpubic disc
Adductor longus muscle
Deferent duct
Testicular artery
Arcuate pubic ligament
Dorsal vein of penis
Great saphenous vein
Visceral pelvic fascia and prostatic veins
Obturator externus muscle

Coccyx
Levator ani
Muscular coat of rectum
Rectal columns
Internal pudendal artery and vein
Greater sciatic foramen
Inferior gluteal artery and vein
Sciatic nerve

Prostatic part of urethra
Right lobe of prostate
Median lobe of prostate
Ejaculatory ducts

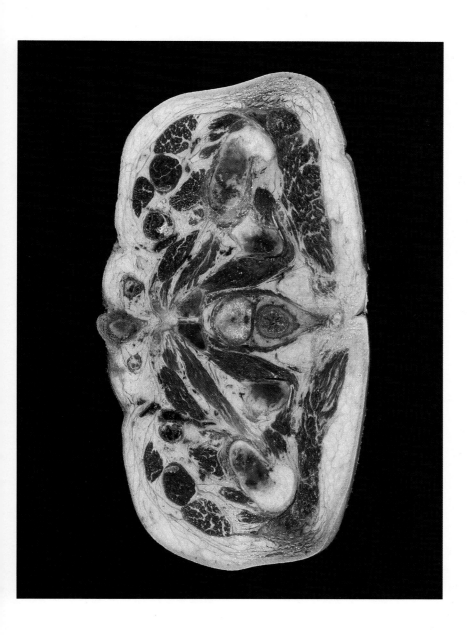

Transverse **Pelvis—Male**

Plate 59

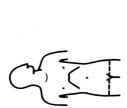

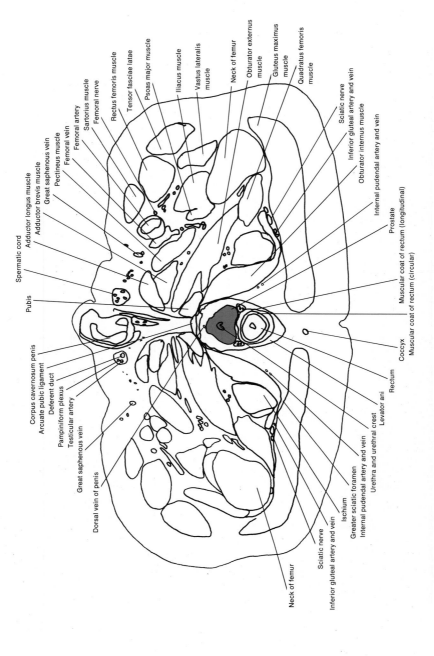

Spermatic cord

Pubis

Corpus cavernosum penis
Arcuate pubic ligament
Deferent duct
Pampiniform plexus
Testicular artery

Great saphenous vein

Dorsal vein of penis

Adductor longus muscle
Adductor brevis muscle
Great saphenous vein
Pectineus muscle
Femoral vein
Sartorius muscle
Femoral nerve
Rectus femoris muscle
Tensor fasciae latae
Psoas major muscle
Femoral artery

Iliacus muscle
Vastus lateralis muscle
Neck of femur
Obturator externus muscle
Gluteus maximus muscle
Quadratus femoris muscle

Sciatic nerve
Inferior gluteal artery and vein
Obturator internus muscle

Internal pudendal artery and vein

Prostate

Muscular coat of rectum (longitudinal)
Muscular coat of rectum (circular)

Coccyx

Rectum

Levator ani
Urethra and urethral crest
Internal pudendal artery and vein
Greater sciatic foramen
Ischium
Inferior gluteal artery and vein
Sciatic nerve

Neck of femur

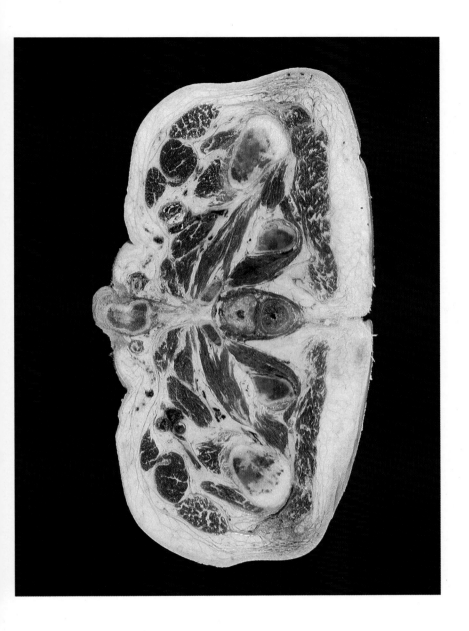

Transverse **Pelvis—Male**

Plate 60

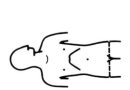

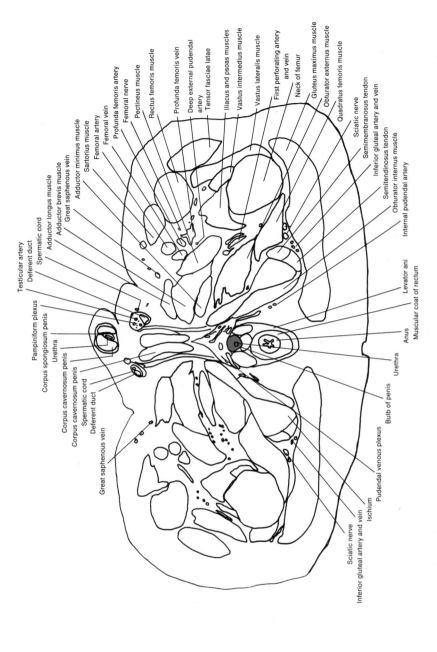

Testicular artery
Deferent duct
Spermatic cord

Pampiniform plexus
Corpus spongiosum penis
Urethra
Corpus cavernosum penis
Corpus cavernosum penis
Spermatic cord
Deferent duct

Great saphenous vein

Adductor longus muscle
Adductor brevis muscle
Great saphenous vein
Adductor minimus muscle
Sartorius muscle
Femoral artery
Femoral vein
Profunda femoris artery
Femoral nerve
Pectineus muscle
Rectus femoris muscle
Profunda femoris vein
Deep external pudendal artery
Tensor fasciae latae
Iliacus and psoas muscles
Vastus intermedius muscle
Vastus lateralis muscle
First perforating artery and vein
Neck of femur
Gluteus maximus muscle
Obturator externus muscle
Quadratus femoris muscle
Sciatic nerve
Semimembranosus tendon
Inferior gluteal artery and vein
Semitendinosus tendon
Obturator internus muscle
Internal pudendal artery

Anus
Muscular coat of rectum

Levator ani

Urethra

Bulb of penis

Pudendal venous plexus

Ischium

Inferior gluteal artery and vein

Sciatic nerve

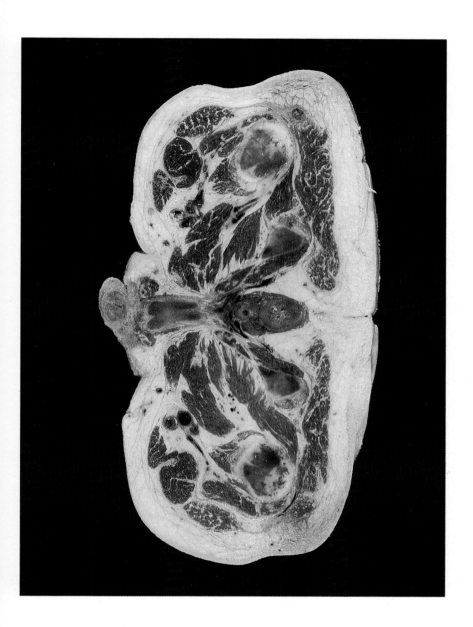

Plate 61

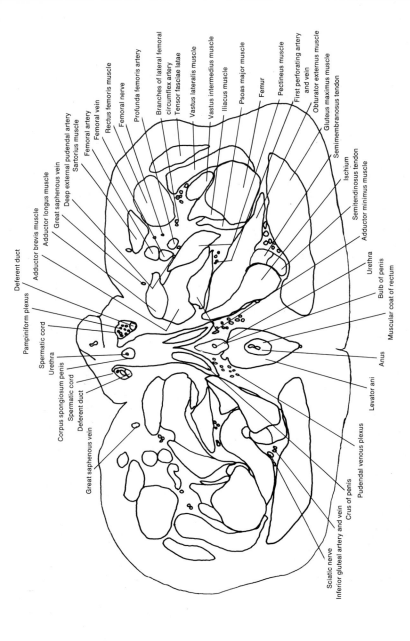

Deferent duct
Adductor brevis muscle
Adductor longus muscle
Great saphenous vein
Deep external pudendal artery
Sartorius muscle
Femoral artery
Femoral vein
Rectus femoris muscle
Femoral nerve
Profunda femoris artery
Branches of lateral femoral circumflex artery
Tensor fasciae latae
Vastus lateralis muscle
Vastus intermedius muscle
Iliacus muscle
Psoas major muscle
Femur
Pectineus muscle
First perforating artery and vein
Obturator externus muscle
Gluteus maximus tendon
Semimembranosus tendon
Semitendinosus tendon
Ischium
Adductor minimus muscle

Pampiniform plexus
Spermatic cord
Urethra
Corpus spongiosum penis
Spermatic cord
Deferent duct
Great saphenous vein

Sciatic nerve
Inferior gluteal artery and vein
Crus of penis
Pudendal venous plexus
Levator ani
Anus
Muscular coat of rectum
Bulb of penis
Urethra

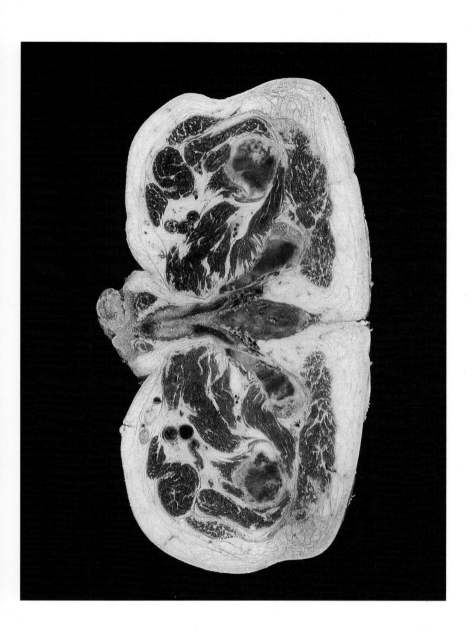

Transverse **Pelvis—Male**

Plate 62

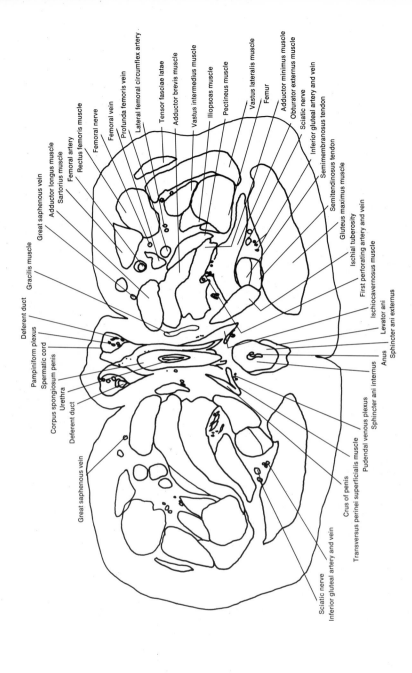

Deferent duct
Gracilis muscle
Great saphenous vein
Adductor longus muscle
Sartorius muscle
Femoral artery
Rectus femoris muscle
Femoral nerve
Femoral vein
Profunda femoris vein
Lateral femoral circumflex artery
Tensor fasciae latae
Adductor brevis muscle
Vastus intermedius muscle
Iliopsoas muscle
Pectineus muscle
Vastus lateralis muscle
Femur
Adductor minimus muscle
Obturator externus muscle
Sciatic nerve
Inferior gluteal artery and vein
Semimembranosus tendon
Semitendinosus muscle
Gluteus maximus muscle
Ischial tuberosity
First perforating artery and vein
Ischiocavernosus muscle
Levator ani
Anus
Sphincter ani externus

Pampiniform plexus
Spermatic cord
Corpus spongiosum penis
Urethra
Deferent duct

Sphincter ani internus
Pudendal venous plexus
Transversus perinei superficialis muscle
Crus of penis

Great saphenous vein

Sciatic nerve
Inferior gluteal artery and vein

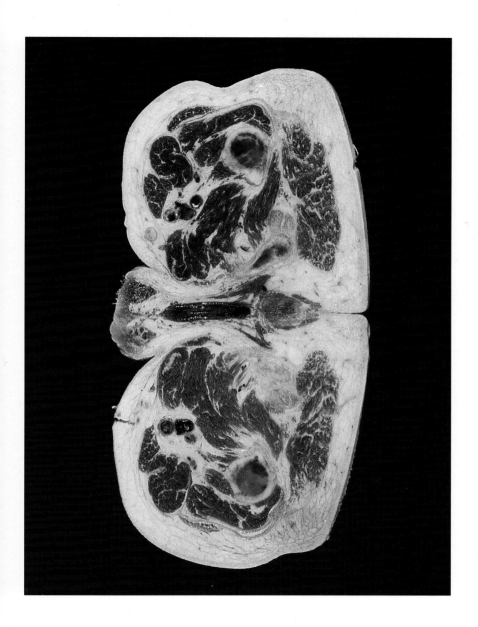

Plate 63

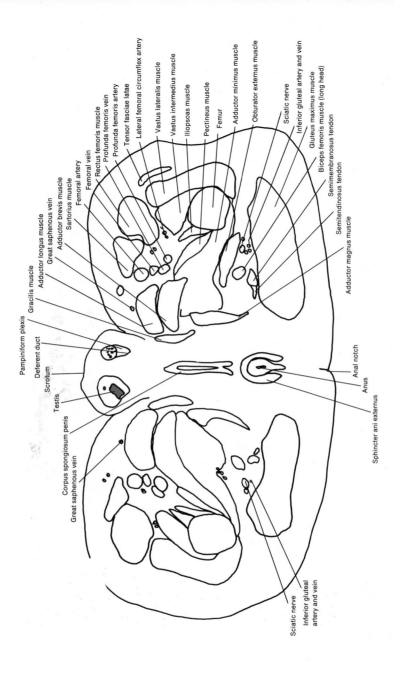

Pampiniform plexis
Deferent duct
Scrotum
Testis
Gracilis muscle
Adductor longus muscle
Adductor brevis muscle
Sartorius muscle
Great saphenous vein
Femoral artery
Femoral vein
Rectus femoris muscle
Profunda femoris vein
Profunda femoris artery
Tensor fasciae latae
Lateral femoral circumflex artery
Vastus lateralis muscle
Vastus intermedius muscle
Iliopsoas muscle
Pectineus muscle
Femur
Adductor minimus muscle
Obturator externus muscle
Sciatic nerve
Inferior gluteal artery and vein
Gluteus maximus muscle
Biceps femoris muscle (long head)
Semimembranosus tendon
Semitendinosus tendon
Adductor magnus muscle

Corpus spongiosum penis
Great saphenous vein

Anal notch
Anus

Sphincter ani externus

Sciatic nerve
Inferior gluteal artery and vein

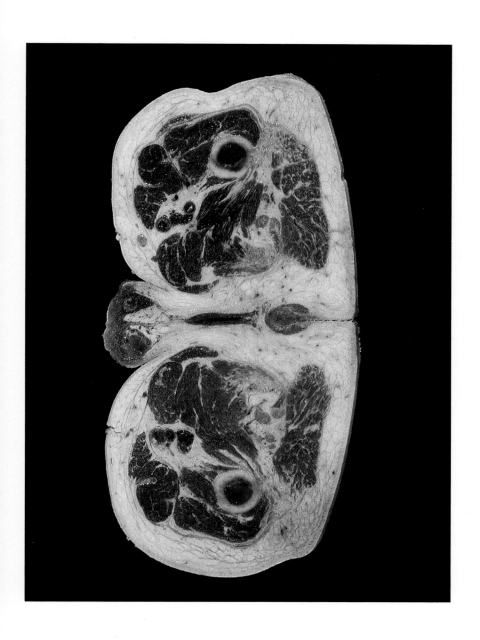

Transverse **Pelvis—Male**

Plate 64

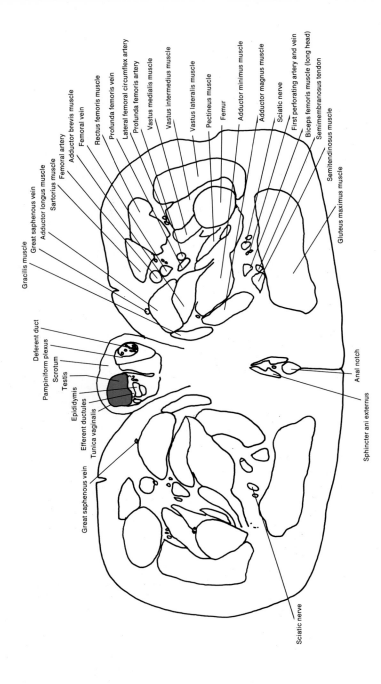

Gracilis muscle
Great saphenous vein
Adductor longus muscle
Sartorius muscle
Femoral artery
Adductor brevis muscle
Femoral vein
Rectus femoris muscle
Profunda femoris vein
Lateral femoral circumflex artery
Profunda femoris artery
Vastus medialis muscle
Vastus intermedius muscle
Vastus lateralis muscle
Pectineus muscle
Femur
Adductor minimus muscle
Adductor magnus muscle
Sciatic nerve
First perforating artery and vein
Biceps femoris muscle (long head)
Semimembranosus tendon
Semitendinosus muscle
Gluteus maximus muscle

Deferent duct
Pampiniform plexus
Scrotum
Testis
Epididymis
Efferent ductules
Tunica vaginalis

Great saphenous vein

Anal notch

Sphincter ani externus

Sciatic nerve

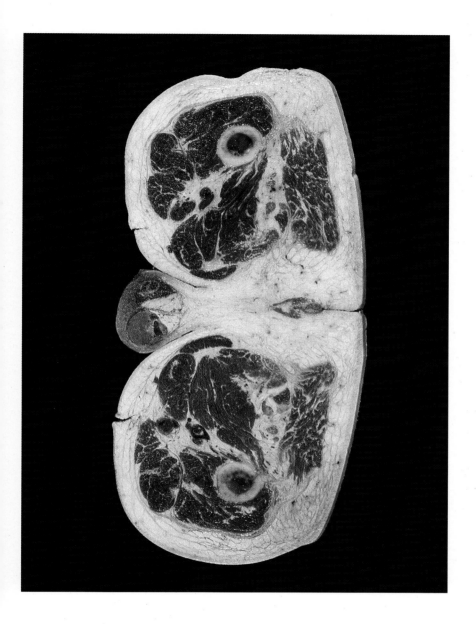

Transverse **Pelvis—Male**

Part Two   PARASAGITTAL SECTIONS

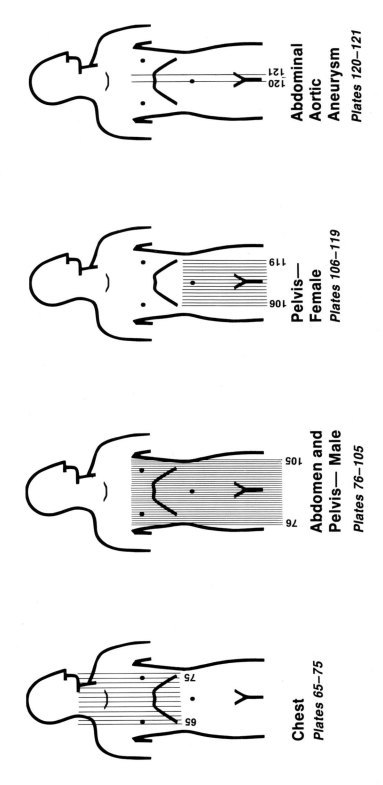

Chest
Plates 65–75

**Abdomen and
Pelvis— Male**
Plates 76–105

**Pelvis—
Female**
Plates 106–119

**Abdominal
Aortic
Aneurysm**
Plates 120–121

PARASAGITTAL   Chest   *Plates 65–75*

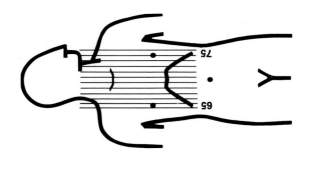

Plate 65

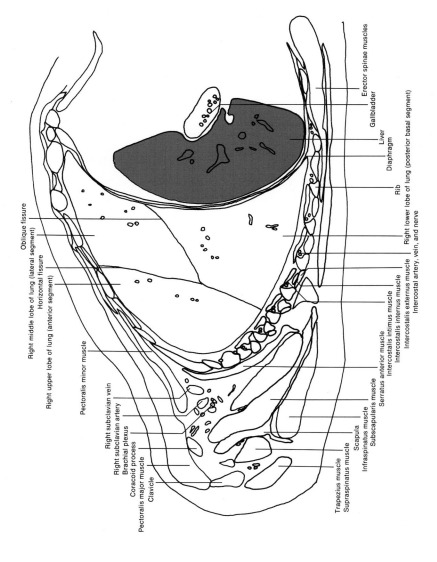

Oblique fissure
Right middle lobe of lung (lateral segment)
Horizontal fissure
Right upper lobe of lung (anterior segment)

Pectoralis minor muscle

Right subclavian vein
Right subclavian artery
Brachial plexus
Coracoid process
Pectoralis major muscle
Clavicle

Trapezius muscle
Supraspinatus muscle
Scapula
Infraspinatus muscle
Subscapularis muscle
Serratus anterior muscle
Intercostalis intimus muscle
Intercostalis internus muscle
Intercostalis externus muscle
Intercostal artery, vein, and nerve

Right lower lobe of lung (posterior basal segment)
Rib
Diaphragm
Liver
Gallbladder
Erector spinae muscles

Parasagittal **Chest**

Plate 66

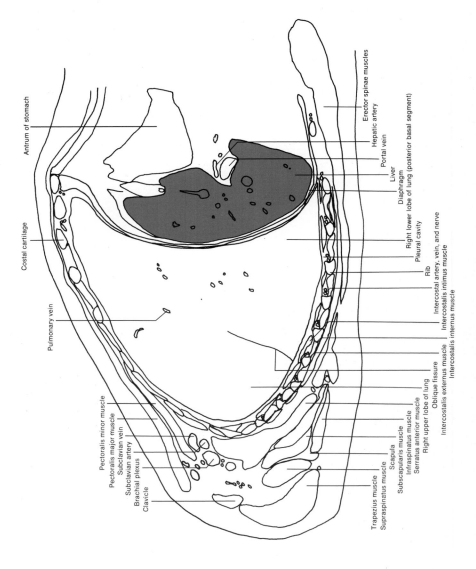

Antrum of stomach

Costal cartilage

Pulmonary vein

Pectoralis minor muscle
Pectoralis major muscle
Subclavian vein
Subclavian artery
Brachial plexus
Clavicle

Trapezius muscle
Supraspinatus muscle
Scapula
Subscapularis muscle
Infraspinatus muscle
Serratus anterior muscle
Right upper lobe of lung
Oblique fissure
Intercostalis externus muscle
Intercostalis internus muscle
Intercostalis intimus muscle
Intercostal artery, vein, and nerve
Rib
Pleural cavity
Right lower lobe of lung (posterior basal segment)
Diaphragm
Liver
Portal vein
Hepatic artery
Erector spinae muscles

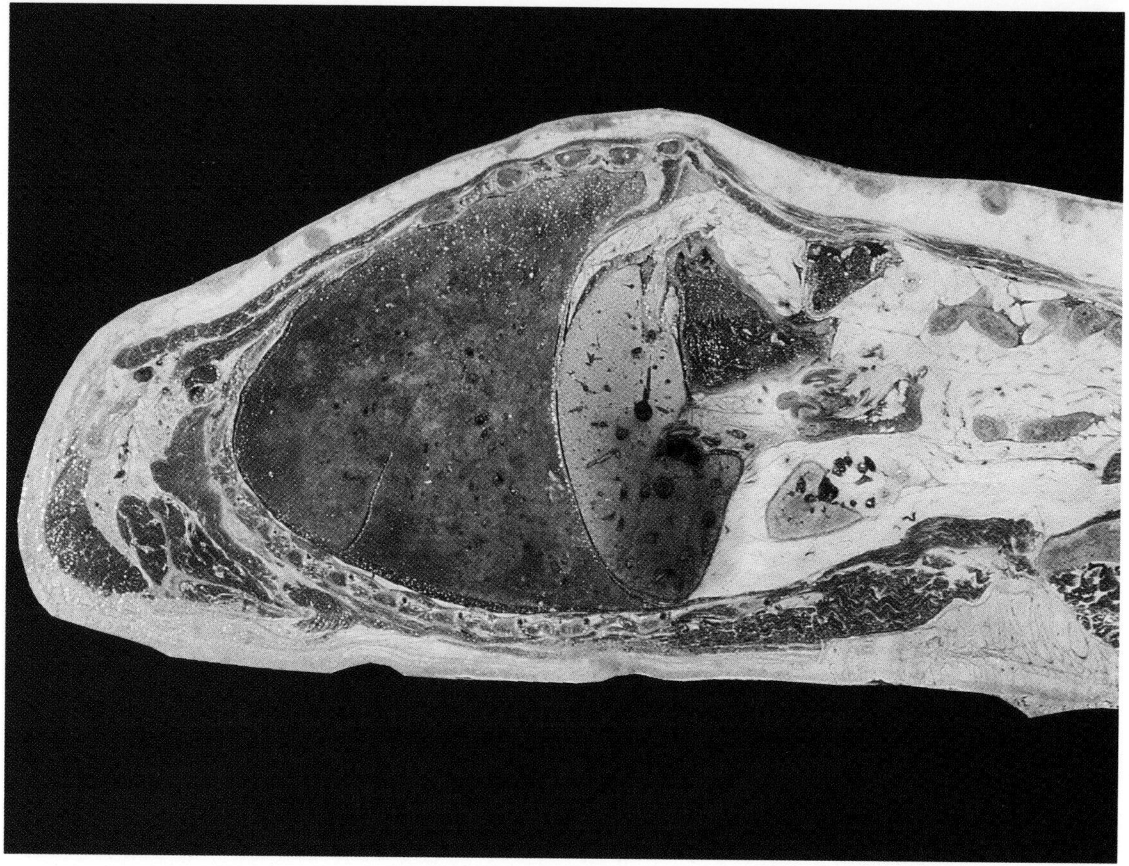

Plate 67

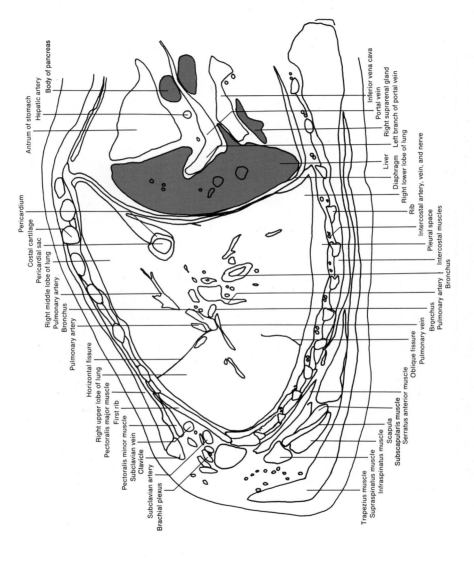

Antrum of stomach
Hepatic artery
Body of pancreas

Inferior vena cava
Portal vein
Right suprarenal gland
Left branch of portal vein
Liver
Diaphragm
Right lower lobe of lung
Rib
Intercostal artery, vein, and nerve
Pleural space
Intercostal muscles

Pericardium
Costal cartilage
Pericardial sac
Right middle lobe of lung
Pulmonary artery
Bronchus
Pulmonary artery

Bronchus
Pulmonary artery
Bronchus
Pulmonary vein
Oblique fissure
Serratus anterior muscle
Subscapularis muscle
Scapula
Infraspinatus muscle
Supraspinatus muscle
Trapezius muscle

Horizontal fissure
Right upper lobe of lung
Pectoralis major muscle
First rib
Pectoralis minor muscle
Subclavian vein
Clavicle
Subclavian artery
Brachial plexus

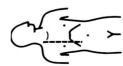

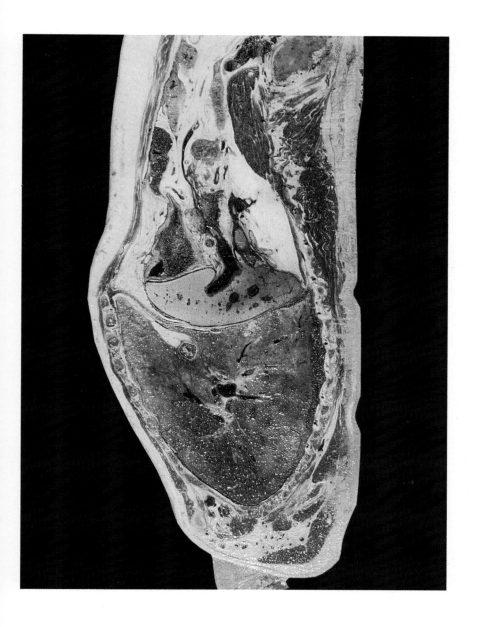

Plate 68

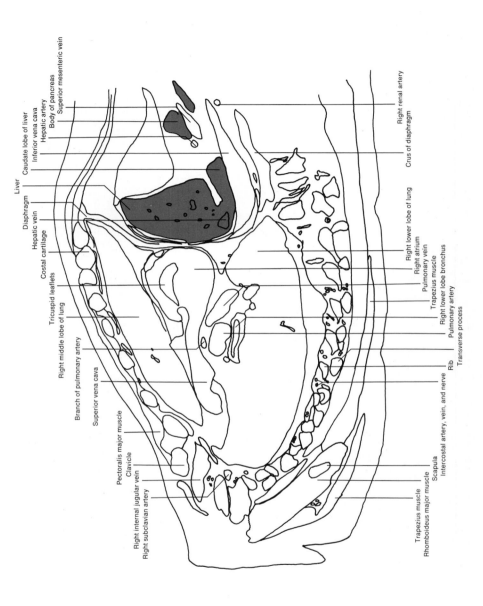
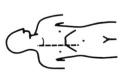

Superior mesenteric vein
Body of pancreas
Hepatic artery
Inferior vena cava
Caudate lobe of liver

Right renal artery

Liver

Crus of diaphragm

Diaphragm
Hepatic vein
Costal cartilage

Tricuspid leaflets

Right lower lobe of lung
Right atrium
Pulmonary vein
Trapezius muscle
Right lower lobe bronchus
Pulmonary artery

Right middle lobe of lung

Branch of pulmonary artery

Rib
Transverse process

Superior vena cava

Intercostal artery, vein, and nerve

Pectoralis major muscle
Clavicle

Scapula

Right internal jugular vein
Right subclavian artery

Trapezius muscle
Rhomboideus major muscle

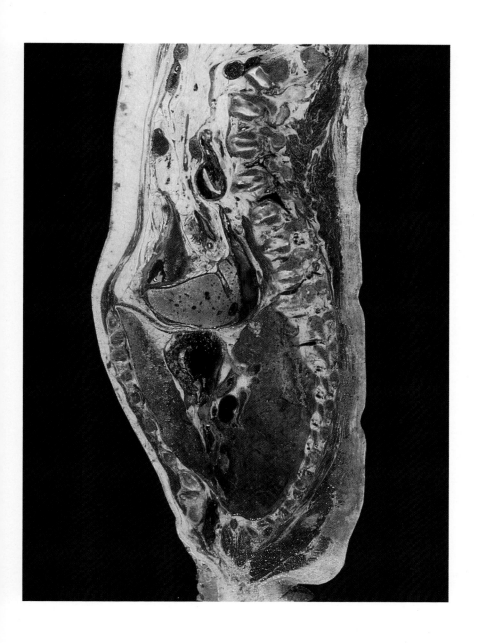

Plate 69

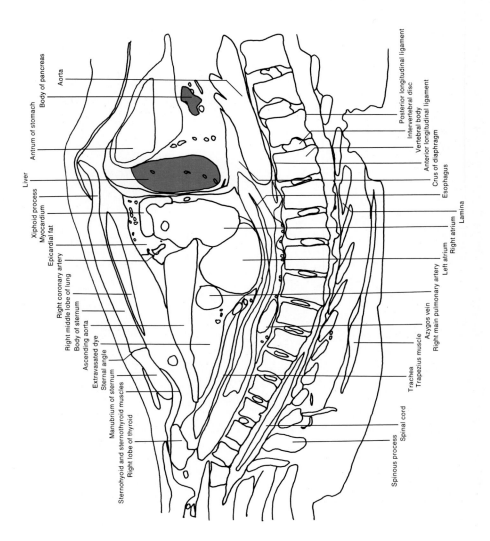

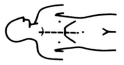

Body of pancreas
Aorta
Antrum of stomach
Liver
Xiphoid process
Myocardium
Epicardial fat
Right coronary artery
Right middle lobe of lung
Body of sternum
Ascending aorta
Extravasated dye
Sternal angle
Manubrium of sternum
Sternohyoid and sternothyroid muscles
Right lobe of thyroid

Posterior longitudinal ligament
Intervertebral disc
Vertebral body
Anterior longitudinal ligament
Crus of diaphragm
Esophagus
Lamina
Right atrium
Left atrium
Right main pulmonary artery
Azygos vein
Trapezius muscle
Trachea
Spinal cord
Spinous process

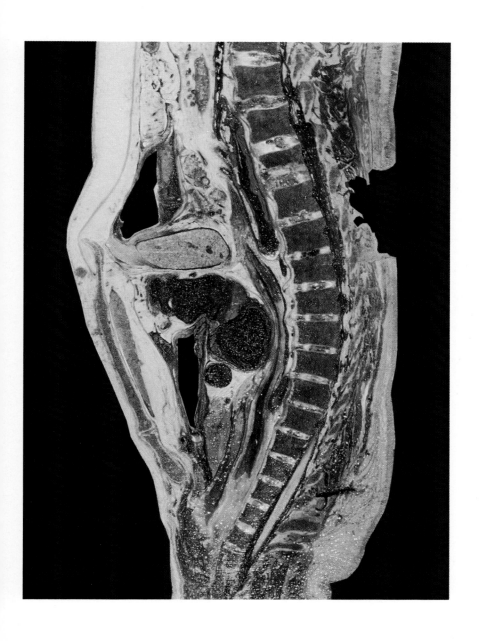

Plate 70

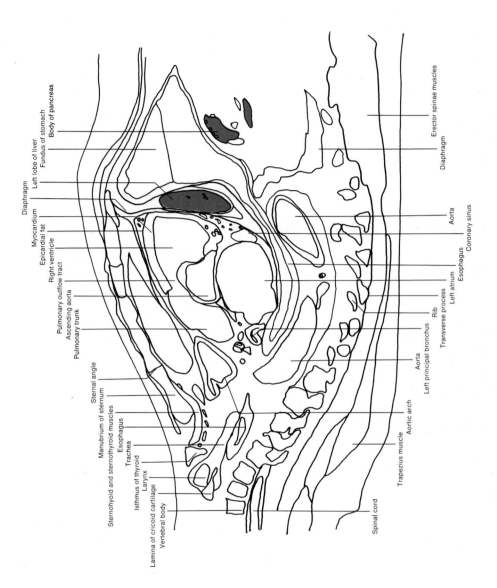

Diaphragm
Left lobe of liver
Fundus of stomach
Body of pancreas

Myocardium
Epicardial fat
Right ventricle
Pulmonary outflow tract
Ascending aorta
Pulmonary trunk

Sternal angle
Manubrium of sternum
Sternohyoid and sternothyroid muscles
Esophagus
Trachea
Isthmus of thyroid
Larynx
Lamina of cricoid cartilage
Vertebral body

Erector spinae muscles

Diaphragm

Aorta
Coronary sinus

Esophagus
Left atrium
Transverse process
Rib
Left principal bronchus
Aorta

Aortic arch

Trapezius muscle

Spinal cord

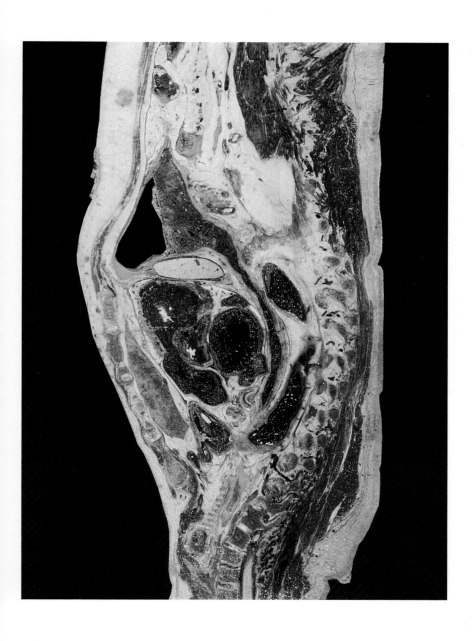

Parasagittal **Chest**

Plate 71

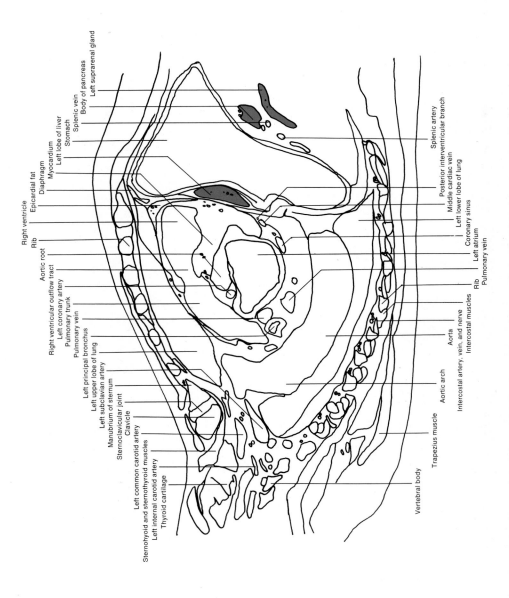

Right ventricle
Rib
Epicardial fat
Diaphragm
Myocardium
Left lobe of liver
Stomach
Splenic vein
Body of pancreas
Left suprarenal gland

Aortic root
Right ventricular outflow tract
Left coronary artery
Pulmonary trunk
Pulmonary vein
Left principal bronchus
Left upper lobe of lung
Left subclavian artery
Manubrium of sternum
Clavicle
Sternoclavicular joint
Left common carotid artery
Sternohyoid and sternothyroid muscles
Left internal carotid artery
Thyroid cartilage

Splenic artery
Posterior interventricular branch
Middle cardiac vein
Left lower lobe of lung
Coronary sinus
Left atrium
Pulmonary vein
Rib
Aorta
Intercostal artery, vein, and nerve
Intercostal muscles

Trapezius muscle

Vertebral body

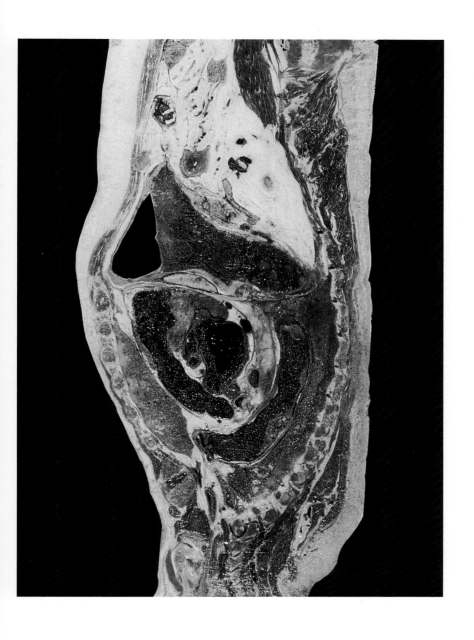

Parasagittal **Chest**

Plate 72

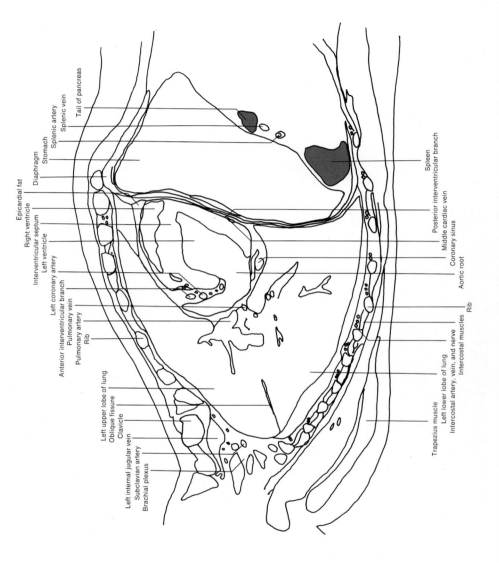

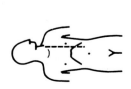

Epicardial fat
Diaphragm
Stomach
Splenic artery
Splenic vein
Tail of pancreas

Right ventricle
Interventricular septum
Left ventricle
Left coronary artery
Anterior interventricular branch
Pulmonary vein
Pulmonary artery
Rib

Left upper lobe of lung
Oblique fissure
Clavicle
Left internal jugular vein
Subclavian artery
Brachial plexus

Spleen
Posterior interventricular branch
Middle cardiac vein
Coronary sinus
Aortic root

Rib
Intercostal muscles
Intercostal artery, vein, and nerve
Left lower lobe of lung
Trapezius muscle

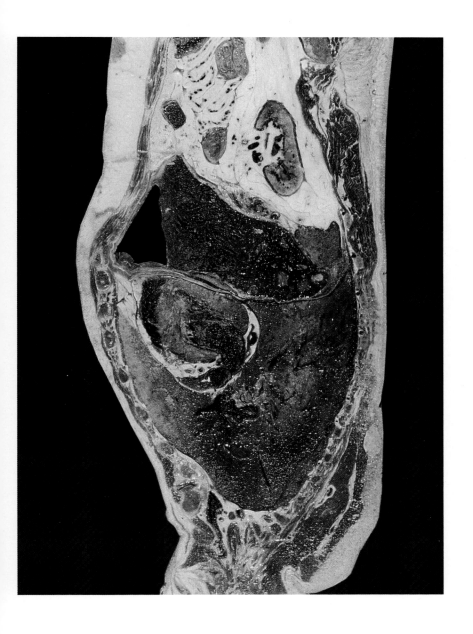

Parasagittal **Chest**

Plate 73

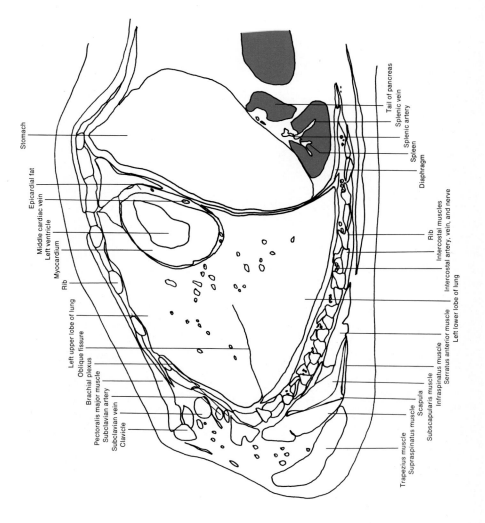

Stomach

Epicardial fat
Middle cardiac vein
Left ventricle
Myocardium
Rib

Left upper lobe of lung
Oblique fissure
Brachial plexus
Pectoralis major muscle
Subclavian artery
Subclavian vein
Clavicle

Tail of pancreas
Splenic vein
Splenic artery
Spleen
Diaphragm

Rib
Intercostal muscles
Intercostal artery, vein, and nerve
Left lower lobe of lung

Serratus anterior muscle
Infraspinatus muscle
Scapula
Subscapularis muscle
Supraspinatus muscle
Trapezius muscle

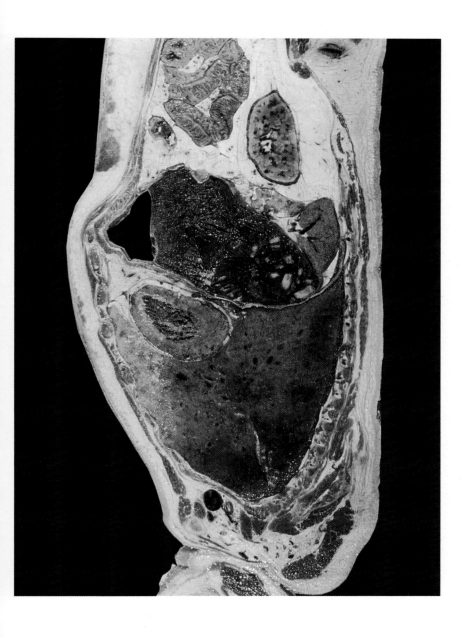

Parasagittal **Chest**

Plate 74

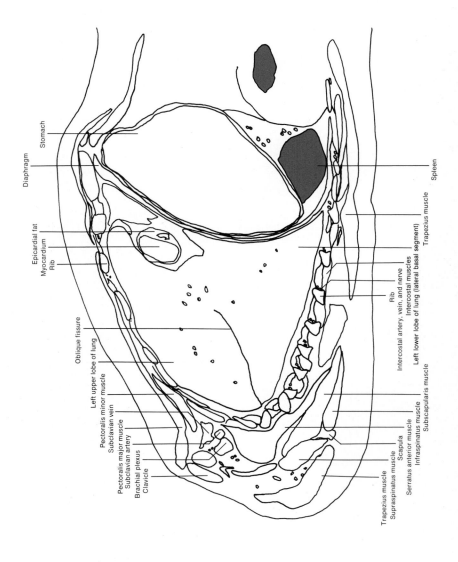

Stomach

Diaphragm

Epicardial fat
Myocardium
Rib

Oblique fissure

Left upper lobe of lung
Pectoralis minor muscle
Subclavian vein
Pectoralis major muscle
Subclavian artery
Brachial plexus
Clavicle

Spleen

Trapezius muscle

Rib
Intercostal artery, vein, and nerve
Intercostal muscles
Left lower lobe of lung (lateral basal segment)

Subscapularis muscle

Trapezius muscle
Supraspinatus muscle
Scapula
Serratus anterior muscle
Infraspinatus muscle

Y

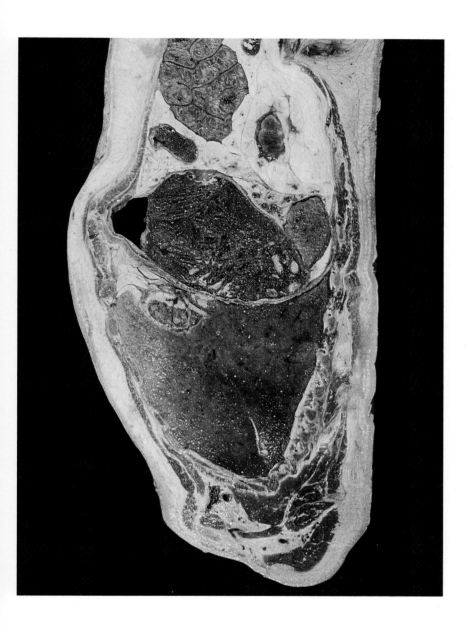

Parasagittal **Chest**

Plate 75

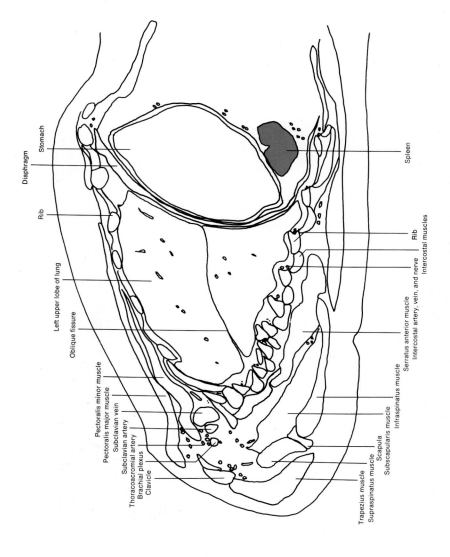

Stomach

Diaphragm

Rib

Left upper lobe of lung

Oblique fissure

Pectoralis minor muscle

Pectoralis major muscle

Subclavian vein

Subclavian artery

Thoracoacromial artery

Brachial plexus

Clavicle

Trapezius muscle

Supraspinatus muscle

Subscapularis muscle

Scapula

Infraspinatus muscle

Serratus anterior muscle

Intercostal artery, vein, and nerve

Intercostal muscles

Rib

Spleen

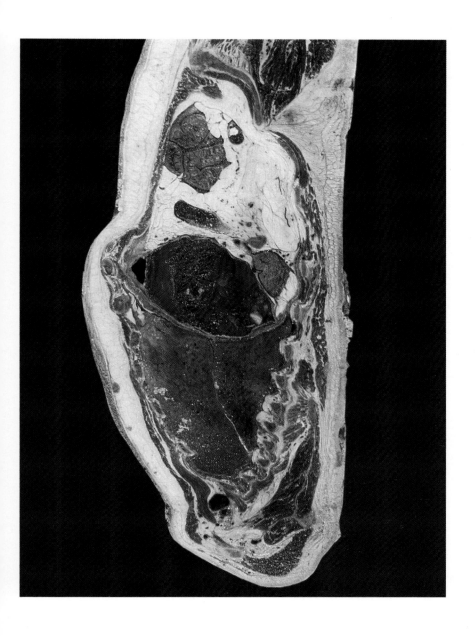

Parasagittal **Chest**

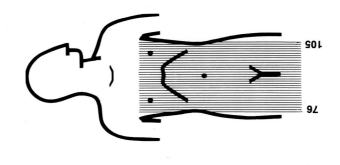

105

76

Hepatic Venous Anatomy

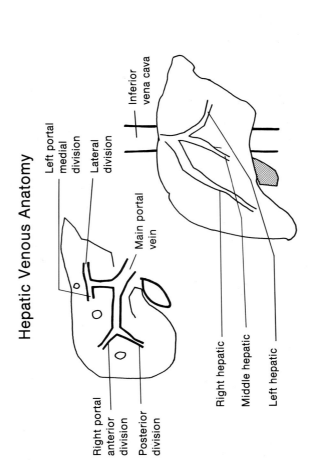

Left portal medial division

Lateral division

Inferior vena cava

Main portal vein

Right portal anterior division

Posterior division

Right hepatic

Middle hepatic

Left hepatic

Plate 76

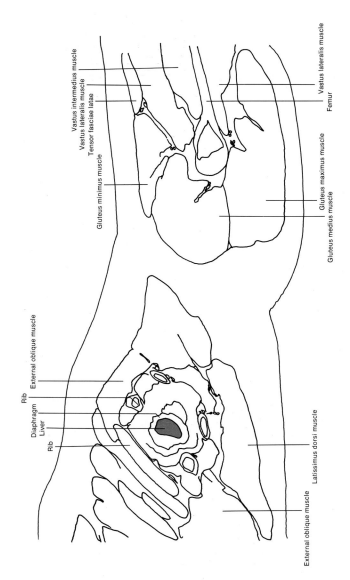

Vastus intermedius muscle

Vastus lateralis muscle

Tensor fasciae latae

Gluteus minimus muscle

Vastus lateralis muscle

Femur

Gluteus maximus muscle

Gluteus medius muscle

External oblique muscle

Rib

Diaphragm

Liver

Rib

Latissimus dorsi muscle

External oblique muscle

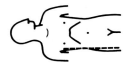

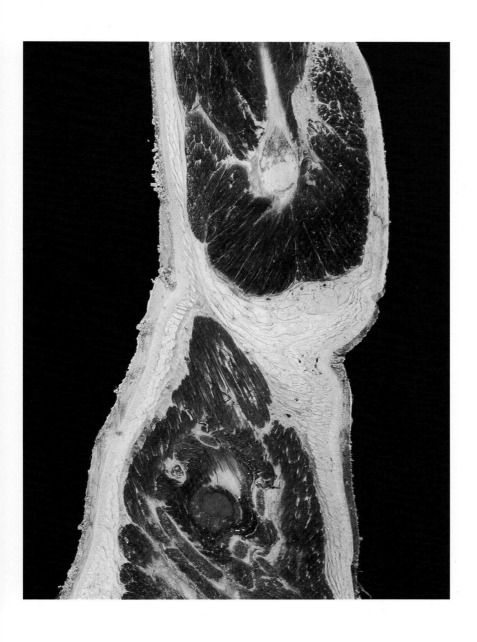

Parasagittal **Abdomen and Pelvis—Male**

Plate 77

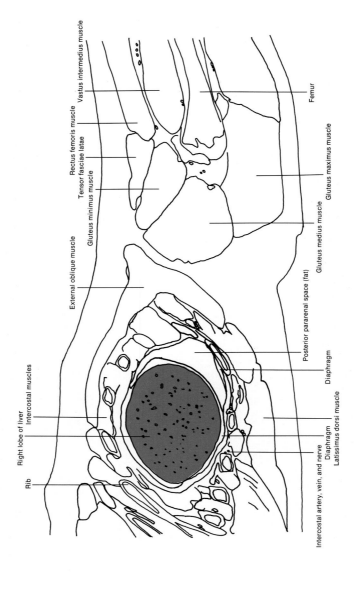

Vastus intermedius muscle

Rectus femoris muscle

Tensor fasciae latae

Gluteus minimus muscle

External oblique muscle

Femur

Gluteus maximus muscle

Gluteus medius muscle

Posterior pararenal space (fat)

Diaphragm

Right lobe of liver

Intercostal muscles

Rib

Intercostal artery, vein, and nerve

Diaphragm

Latissimus dorsi muscle

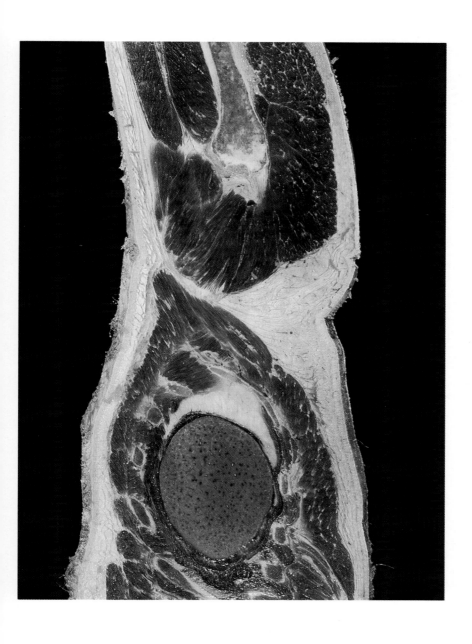

Parasagittal **Abdomen and Pelvis—Male**

Plate 78

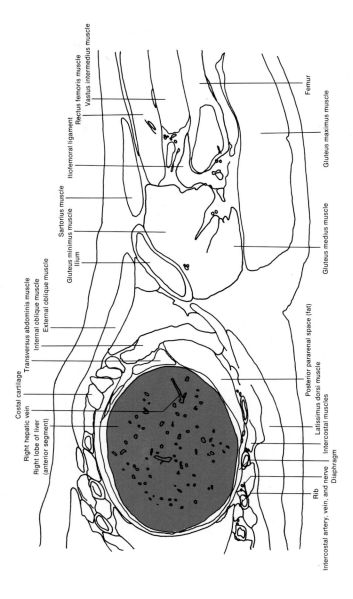

Rectus femoris muscle

Vastus intermedius muscle

Iliofemoral ligament

Sartorius muscle

Gluteus minimus muscle

Ilium

Femur

Gluteus maximus muscle

Gluteus medius muscle

Transversus abdominis muscle

Internal oblique muscle

External oblique muscle

Costal cartilage

Right hepatic vein

Right lobe of liver (anterior segment)

Posterior pararenal space (fat)

Latissimus dorsi muscle

Intercostal muscles

Diaphragm

Rib

Intercostal artery, vein, and nerve

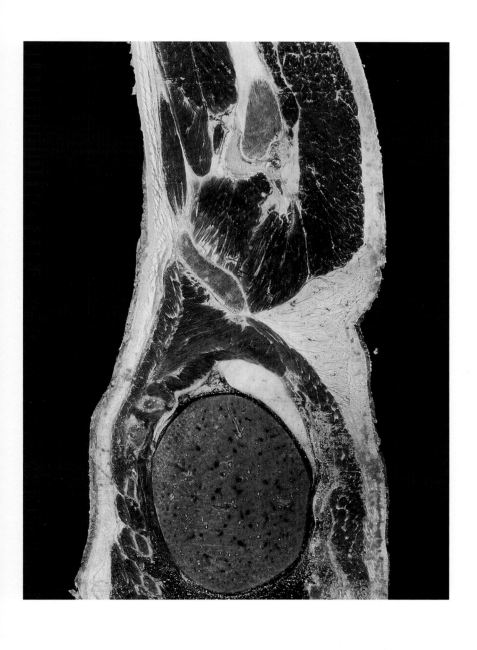

Parasagittal **Abdomen and Pelvis—Male**

Plate 79

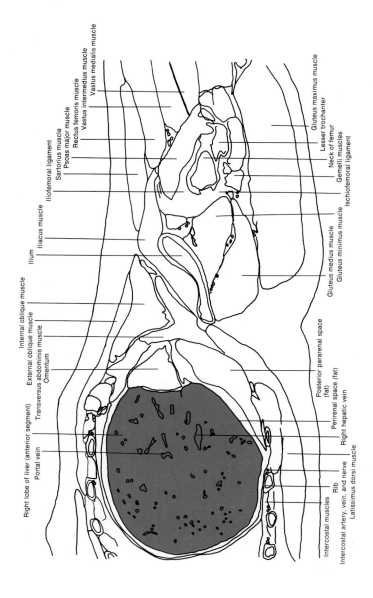

Right lobe of liver (anterior segment)
Portal vein

Internal oblique muscle
External oblique muscle
Transversus abdominis muscle
Omentum

Iliofemoral ligament
Sartorius muscle
Psoas major muscle
Rectus femoris muscle
Vastus intermedius muscle
Vastus medialis muscle

Ilium
Iliacus muscle

Gluteus maximus muscle

Lesser trochanter
Neck of femur
Gemelli muscles
Ischiofemoral ligament

Gluteus medius muscle
Gluteus minimus muscle

Posterior pararenal space
Perirenal space (fat)
Right hepatic vein

Intercostal muscles
Rib
Intercostal artery, vein, and nerve
Latissimus dorsi muscle

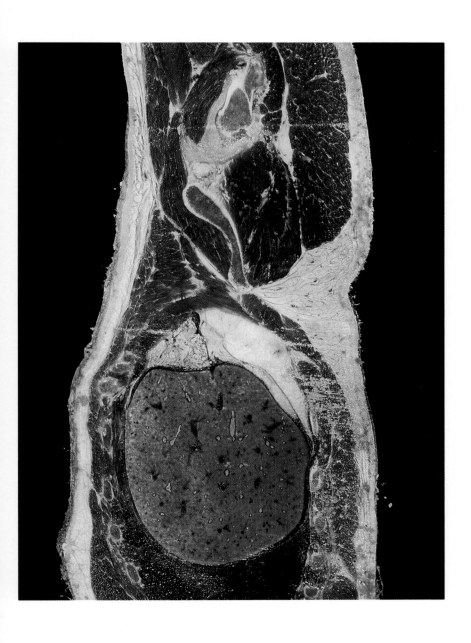

Parasagittal **Abdomen and Pelvis—Male**

Plate 80

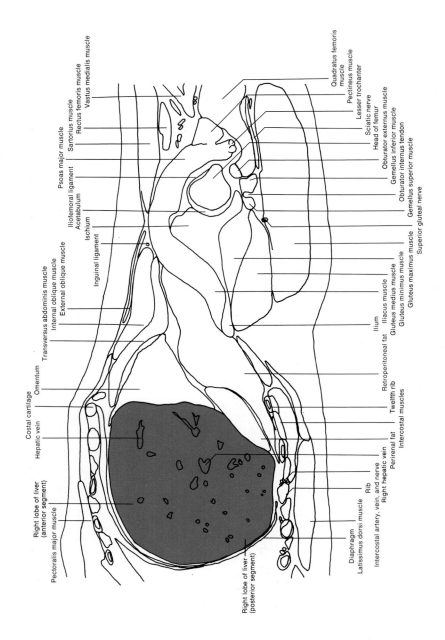

Quadratus femoris muscle
Pectineus muscle
Lesser trochanter
Sciatic nerve
Head of femur
Obturator externus muscle
Gemellus inferior muscle
Obturator internus tendon
Gemellus superior muscle
Superior gluteal nerve

Vastus medialis muscle
Rectus femoris muscle
Sartorius muscle
Psoas major muscle
Iliofemoral ligament
Acetabulum
Ischium
Inguinal ligament

Transversus abdominis muscle
Internal oblique muscle
External oblique muscle
Omentum
Costal cartilage
Hepatic vein

Right lobe of liver
(anterior segment)
Pectoralis major muscle

Right lobe of liver
(posterior segment)

Diaphragm
Latissimus dorsi muscle
Rib
Right hepatic vein
Intercostal artery, vein, and nerve
Perirenal fat
Intercostal muscles
Twelfth rib
Retroperitoneal fat

Ilium
Iliacus muscle
Gluteus medius muscle
Gluteus minimus muscle
Gluteus maximus muscle

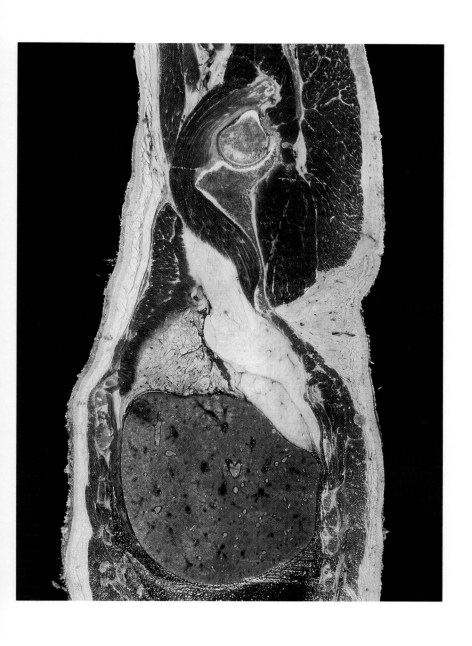

Parasagittal **Abdomen and Pelvis—Male**

Plate 81

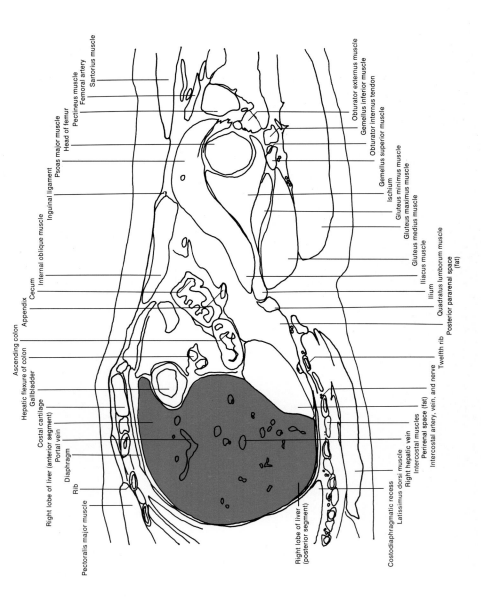

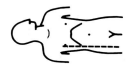

Pectoralis major muscle

Rib

Diaphragm

Right lobe of liver (anterior segment)

Portal vein

Costal cartilage

Gallbladder

Hepatic flexure of colon

Ascending colon

Appendix

Cecum

Internal oblique muscle

Inguinal ligament

Psoas major muscle

Head of femur

Pectineus muscle

Femoral artery

Sartorius muscle

Obturator externus muscle

Gemellus inferior muscle

Obturator internus tendon

Gemellus superior muscle

Ischium

Gluteus minimus muscle

Gluteus maximus muscle

Gluteus medius muscle

Iliacus muscle

Ilium

Quadratus lumborum muscle

Posterior pararenal space (fat)

Twelfth rib

Intercostal artery, vein, and nerve

Perirenal space (fat)

Intercostal muscles

Right hepatic vein

Latissimus dorsi muscle

Costodiaphragmatic recess

Right lobe of liver (posterior segment)

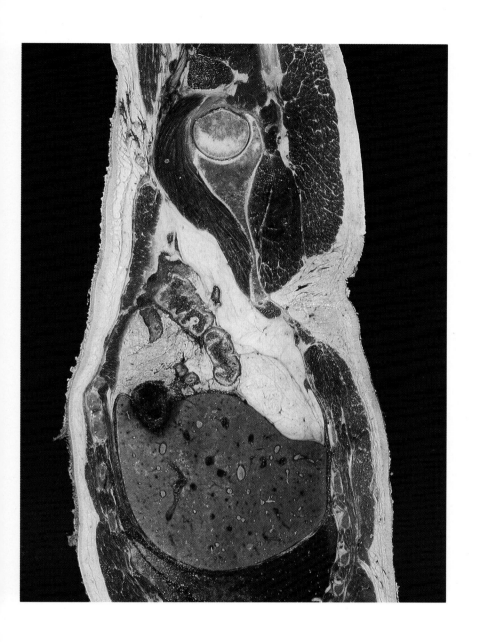

Plate 82

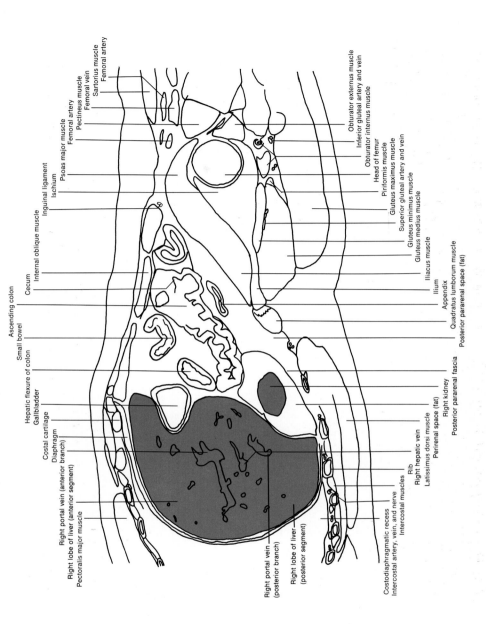

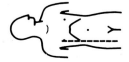

Sartorius muscle
Pectineus muscle
Femoral vein
Femoral artery

Psoas major muscle
Ischium
Inguinal ligament
Internal oblique muscle

Cecum
Ascending colon
Small bowel
Hepatic flexure of colon
Gallbladder

Costal cartilage
Diaphragm

Right portal vein (anterior branch)
Right lobe of liver (anterior segment)
Pectoralis major muscle

Right portal vein (posterior branch)
Right lobe of liver (posterior segment)

Costodiaphragmatic recess
Intercostal artery, vein, and nerve
Intercostal muscles

Rib
Right hepatic vein
Latissimus dorsi muscle

Perirenal space (fat)
Right kidney
Posterior pararenal fascia

Femoral artery
Obturator externus muscle
Inferior gluteal artery and vein
Obturator internus muscle

Head of femur
Piriformis muscle
Gluteus maximus muscle
Superior gluteal artery and vein
Gluteus minimus muscle
Gluteus medius muscle

Iliacus muscle
Ilium
Appendix
Quadratus lumborum muscle
Posterior pararenal space (fat)

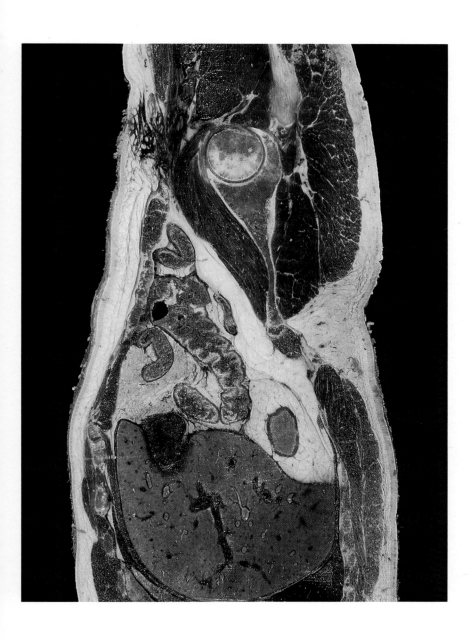

Parasagittal **Abdomen and Pelvis—Male**

Plate 83

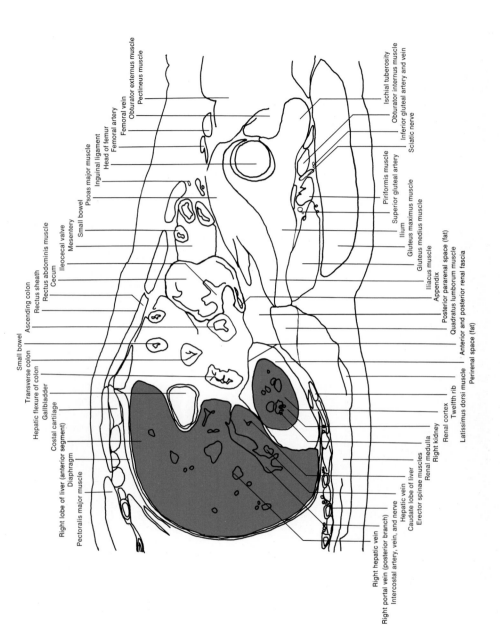

Small bowel
Ascending colon
Rectus sheath
Rectus abdominis muscle
Cecum
Ileocecal valve
Mesentery
Small bowel

Transverse colon
Hepatic flexure of colon
Gallbladder
Costal cartilage
Right lobe of liver (anterior segment)
Diaphragm
Pectoralis major muscle

Obturator externus muscle
Pectineus muscle
Femoral vein
Femoral artery
Head of femur
Inguinal ligament
Psoas major muscle

Ischial tuberosity
Obturator internus muscle
Inferior gluteal artery and vein
Sciatic nerve

Piriformis muscle
Superior gluteal artery
Ilium
Gluteus maximus muscle
Gluteus medius muscle
Iliacus muscle
Appendix
Posterior pararenal space (fat)
Quadratus lumborum muscle
Anterior and posterior renal fascia
Perirenal space (fat)

Right hepatic vein
Right portal vein (posterior branch)
Intercostal artery, vein, and nerve
Hepatic vein
Caudate lobe of liver
Erector spinae muscles
Renal medulla
Right kidney
Renal cortex
Twelfth rib
Latissimus dorsi muscle

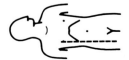

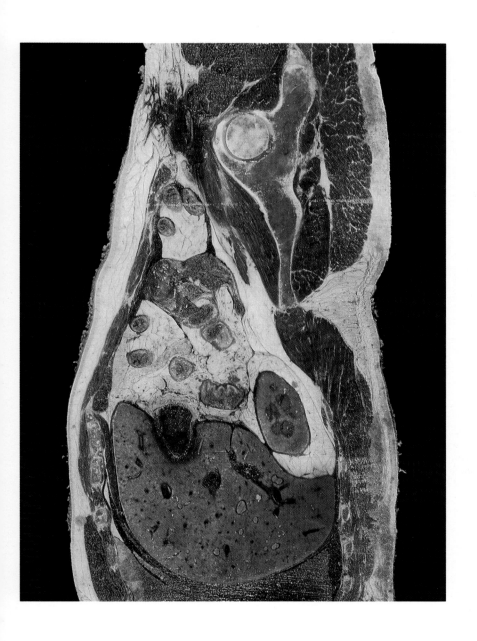

Parasagittal **Abdomen and Pelvis—Male**

Plate 84

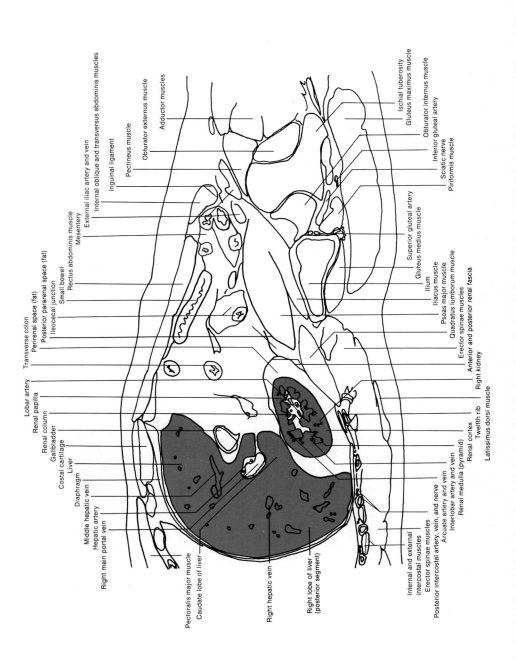

Transverse colon
Perirenal space (fat)
Posterior pararenal space (fat)
Ileocecal junction
Small bowel
Rectus abdominis muscle
Mesentery
External iliac artery and vein
Internal oblique and transversus abdominis muscles
Inguinal ligament
Pectineus muscle
Obturator externus muscle
Adductor muscles

Ischial tuberosity
Gluteus maximus muscle
Obturator internus muscle
Inferior gluteal artery
Sciatic nerve
Piriformis muscle
Superior gluteal artery
Gluteus medius muscle
Ilium
Iliacus muscle
Psoas major muscle
Quadratus lumborum muscle
Erector spinae muscles
Anterior and posterior renal fascia
Right kidney

Lobar artery
Renal papilla
Renal column
Gallbladder
Costal cartilage
Liver
Diaphragm
Middle hepatic vein
Hepatic artery
Right main portal vein

Renal cortex
Twelfth rib
Latissimus dorsi muscle
Internal and external intercostal muscles
Erector spinae muscles
Posterior intercostal artery, vein, and nerve
Arcuate artery and vein
Interlobar artery and vein
Renal medulla (pyramid)

Pectoralis major muscle
Caudate lobe of liver

Right hepatic vein

Right lobe of liver (posterior segment)

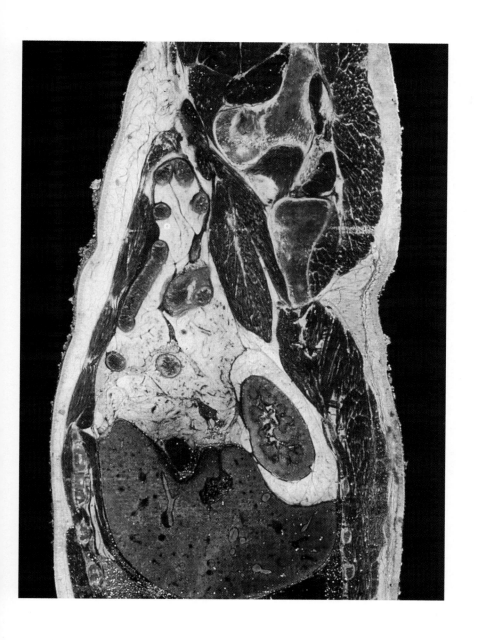

Parasagittal **Abdomen and Pelvis—Male**

Plate 85

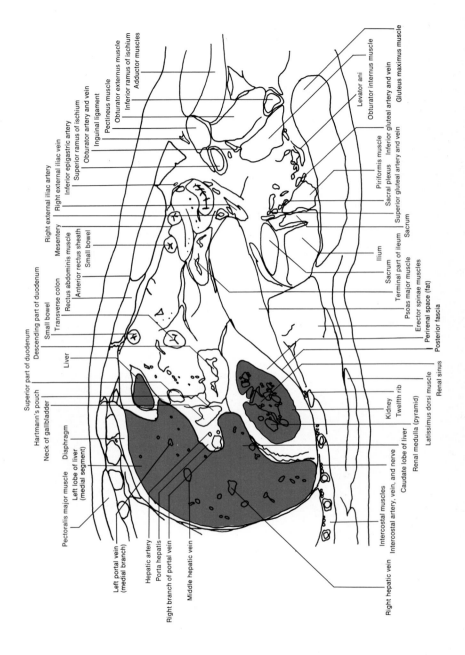

Left portal vein (medial branch)
Hepatic artery
Porta hepatis
Right branch of portal vein
Middle hepatic vein

Pectoralis major muscle
Left lobe of liver (medial segment)
Diaphragm
Neck of gallbladder
Hartmann's pouch
Superior part of duodenum
Descending part of duodenum
Small bowel
Transverse colon
Rectus abdominis muscle
Anterior rectus sheath
Small bowel
Liver
Mesentery
Right external iliac artery
Right external iliac vein
Inferior epigastric artery
Superior ramus of ischium
Obturator artery and vein
Obturator externus muscle
Pectineus muscle
Inguinal ligament
Inferior ramus of ischium
Adductor muscles

Levator ani
Obturator internus muscle
Gluteus maximus muscle
Inferior gluteal artery and vein
Superior gluteal artery and vein
Sacral plexus
Piriformis muscle
Sacrum
Sacrum
Terminal part of ileum
Ilium
Psoas major muscle
Erector spinae muscles
Perirenal space (fat)
Posterior fascia

Renal sinus
Latissimus dorsi muscle
Renal medulla (pyramid)
Caudate lobe of liver
Twelfth rib
Kidney
Intercostal artery, vein, and nerve
Intercostal muscles
Right hepatic vein

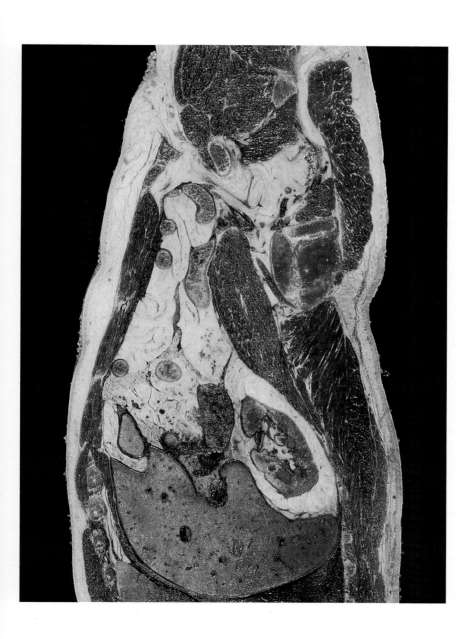

Parasagittal **Abdomen and Pelvis—Male**

Plate 86

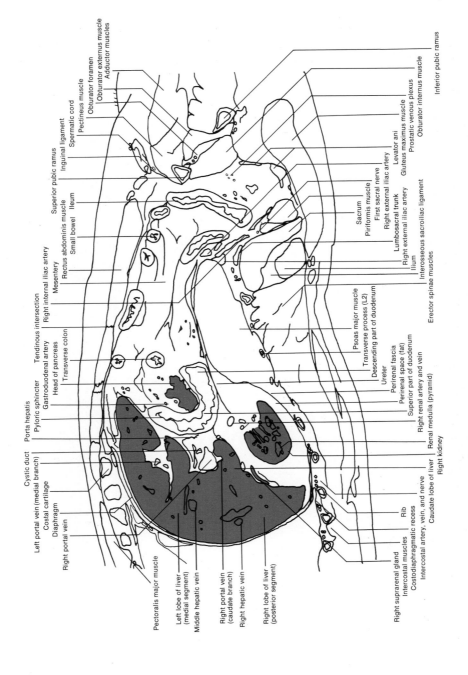

Cystic duct
Porta hepatis
Left portal vein (medial branch)
Costal cartilage
Pyloric sphincter
Tendinous intersection
Diaphragm
Gastroduodenal artery
Right internal iliac artery
Right portal vein
Head of pancreas
Mesentery
Superior pubic ramus
Transverse colon
Rectus abdominis muscle
Inguinal ligament
Small bowel
Ileum
Spermatic cord
Pectineus muscle
Obturator foramen
Obturator externus muscle
Adductor muscles

Pectoralis major muscle
Left lobe of liver (medial segment)
Middle hepatic vein
Right portal vein (caudate branch)
Right hepatic vein
Right lobe of liver (posterior segment)
Caudate lobe of liver
Right kidney
Right suprarenal gland
Intercostal muscles
Costodiaphragmatic recess
Intercostal artery, vein, and nerve
Rib

Psoas major muscle
Transverse process (L2)
Descending part of duodenum
Ureter
Perirenal fascia
Perirenal space (fat)
Superior part of duodenum
Right renal artery and vein
Renal medulla (pyramid)

Erector spinae muscles
Interosseous sacroiliac ligament
Ilium
Right external iliac artery
Lumbosacral trunk
First sacral nerve
Piriformis muscle
Sacrum
Right external iliac artery
Levator ani
Gluteus maximus muscle
Prostatic venous plexus
Obturator internus muscle
Inferior pubic ramus

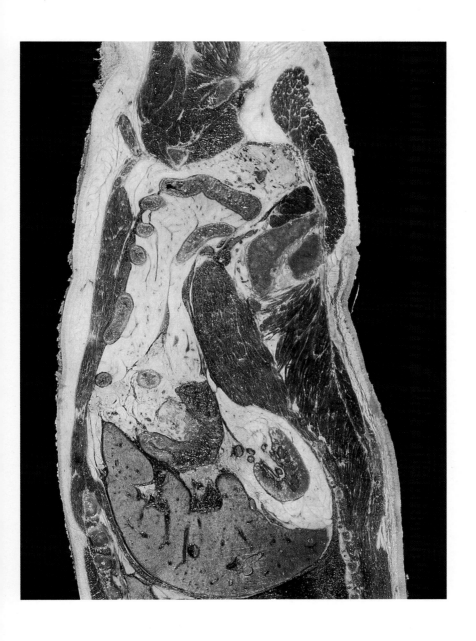

189 Parasagittal **Abdomen and Pelvis—Male**

Plate 87

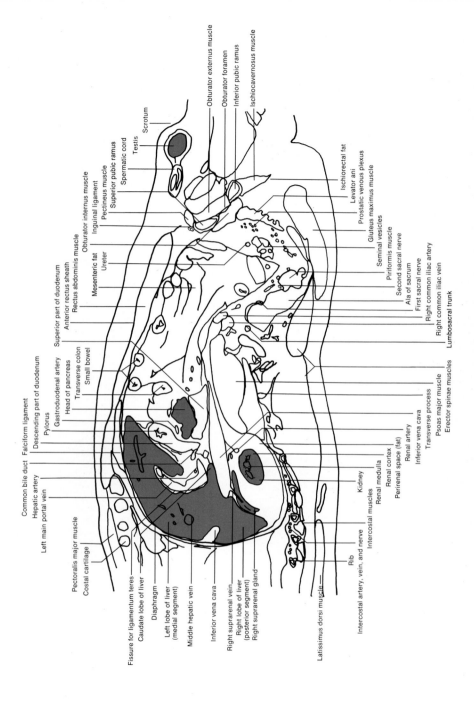

Common bile duct · Falciform ligament
Hepatic artery · Descending part of duodenum
Left main portal vein · Pylorus
Gastroduodenal artery
Head of pancreas
Transverse colon
Small bowel

Superior part of duodenum
Anterior rectus sheath
Rectus abdominis muscle
Mesenteric fat
Ureter
Obturator internus muscle
Inguinal ligament
Pectineus muscle
Superior pubic ramus
Spermatic cord
Testis
Scrotum

Obturator externus muscle
Obturator foramen
Inferior pubic ramus
Ischiocavernosus muscle

Ischiorectal fat
Levator ani
Prostatic venous plexus
Gluteus maximus muscle
Seminal vesicles
Piriformis muscle
Second sacral nerve
Ala of sacrum
First sacral nerve
Right common iliac artery
Right common iliac vein
Lumbosacral trunk

Renal artery
Inferior vena cava
Transverse process
Psoas major muscle
Erector spinae muscles

Pectoralis major muscle
Costal cartilage

Fissure for ligamentum teres
Caudate lobe of liver
Diaphragm
Left lobe of liver
(medial segment)
Middle hepatic vein
Inferior vena cava
Right suprarenal vein
Right lobe of liver
(posterior segment)
Right suprarenal gland

Kidney
Renal medulla
Renal cortex
Perirenal space (fat)

Rib
Intercostal muscles
Intercostal artery, vein, and nerve
Latissimus dorsi muscle

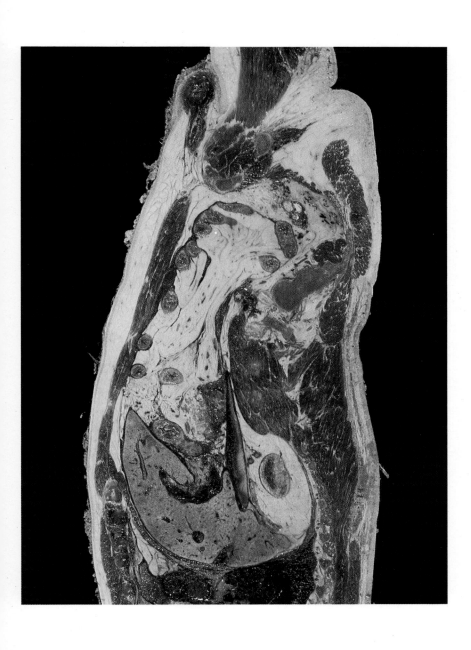

Parasagittal **Abdomen and Pelvis—Male**

Plate 88

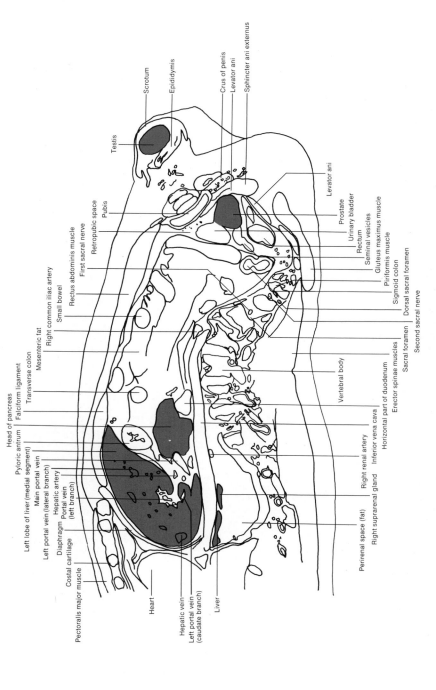

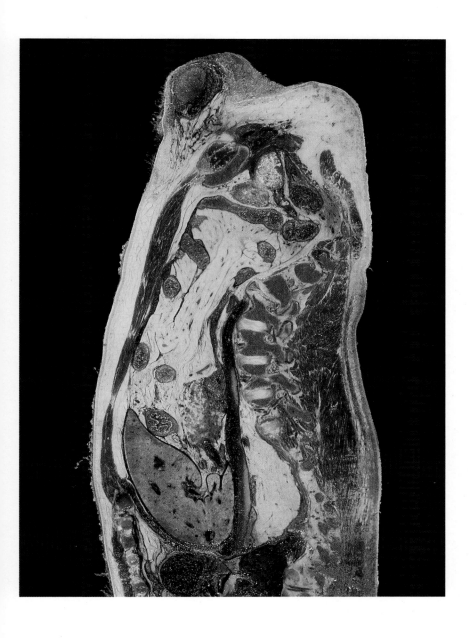

Parasagittal **Abdomen and Pelvis—Male**

Plate 89

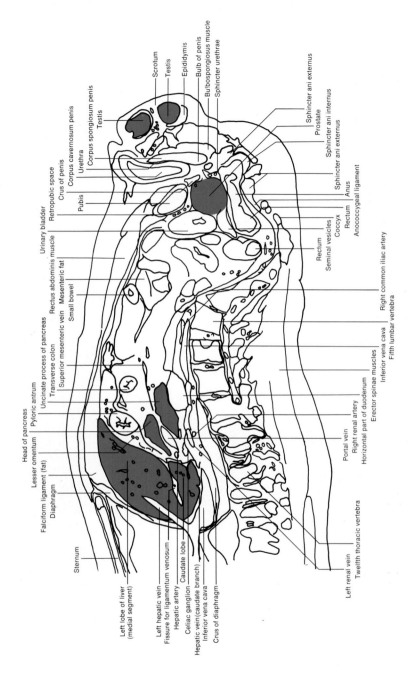

Scrotum
Testis
Epididymis
Bulb of penis
Bulbospongiosus muscle
Sphincter urethrae

Sphincter ani externus
Prostate
Sphincter ani internus
Sphincter ani externus
Anus
Anococcygeal ligament

Rectum
Seminal vesicles
Coccyx
Rectum

Right common iliac artery
Fifth lumbar vertebra
Inferior vena cava
Erector spinae muscles
Horizontal part of duodenum
Right renal artery
Portal vein

Twelfth thoracic vertebra
Left renal vein

Testis
Corpus spongiosum penis
Urethra
Corpus cavernosum penis
Crus of penis
Pubis

Retropubic space
Urinary bladder
Rectus abdominis muscle
Mesenteric fat
Small bowel
Superior mesenteric vein
Transverse colon
Uncinate process of pancreas
Pyloric antrum
Head of pancreas
Lesser omentum
Falciform ligament (fat)
Diaphragm

Sternum

Left lobe of liver
(medial segment)

Left hepatic vein
Fissure for ligamentum venosum
Hepatic artery
Caudate lobe
Celiac ganglion
Hepatic vein (caudate branch)
Inferior vena cava
Crus of diaphragm

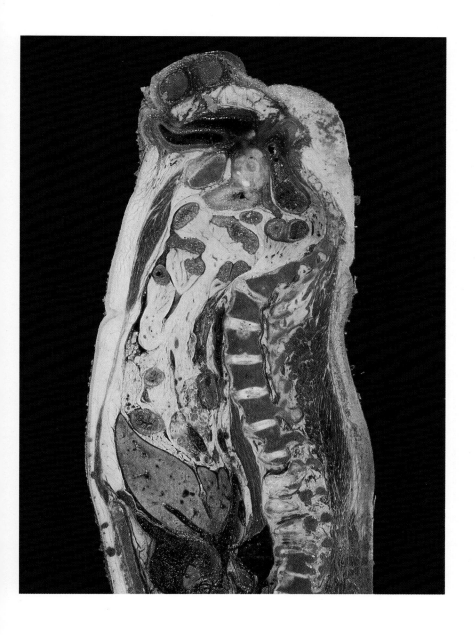

Parasagittal **Abdomen and Pelvis—Male**

Plate 90

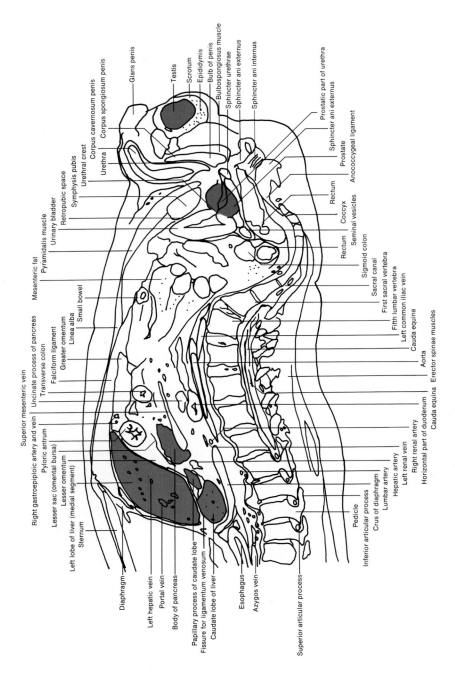

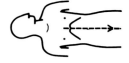

Superior mesenteric vein

Right gastroepiploic artery and vein
Pyloric antrum
Lesser sac (omental bursa)
Lesser omentum
Left lobe of liver (medial segment)
Sternum

Uncinate process of pancreas
Transverse colon

Mesenteric fat

Pyramidalis muscle
Urinary bladder
Retropubic space
Symphysis pubis
Urethral crest
Corpus spongiosum penis
Corpus cavernosum penis
Glans penis

Testis

Scrotum
Epididymis
Bulb of penis
Bulbospongiosus muscle
Sphincter urethrae
Sphincter ani externus
Sphincter ani internus

Prostatic part of urethra

Urethra
Sphincter ani externus
Prostate
Anococcygeal ligament

Rectum
Coccyx
Seminal vesicles

Rectum
Sigmoid colon

Falciform ligament
Greater omentum
Linea alba
Small bowel

Sacral canal
First lumbar vertebra
Fifth lumbar vertebra
Left common iliac vein
Cauda equina
Aorta
Cauda equina
Erector spinae muscles

Diaphragm

Left hepatic vein
Portal vein
Body of pancreas
Papillary process of caudate lobe
Fissure for ligamentum venosum
Caudate lobe of liver
Esophagus
Azygos vein

Superior articular process

Pedicle
Inferior articular process
Crus of diaphragm
Lumbar artery
Hepatic artery
Left renal vein
Right renal artery
Horizontal part of duodenum
Cauda equina

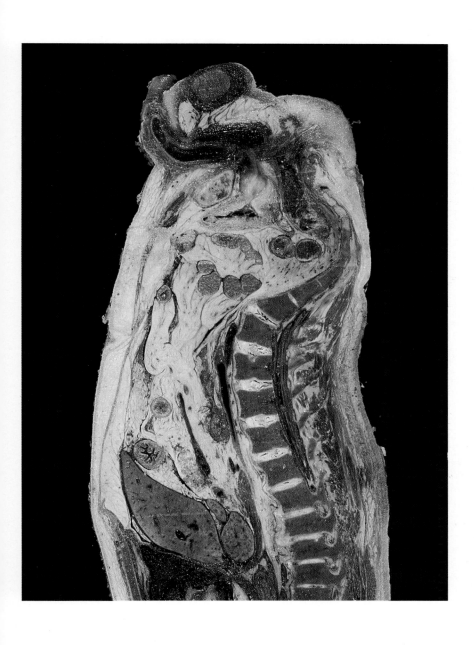

Parasagittal **Abdomen and Pelvis—Male**

Plate 91

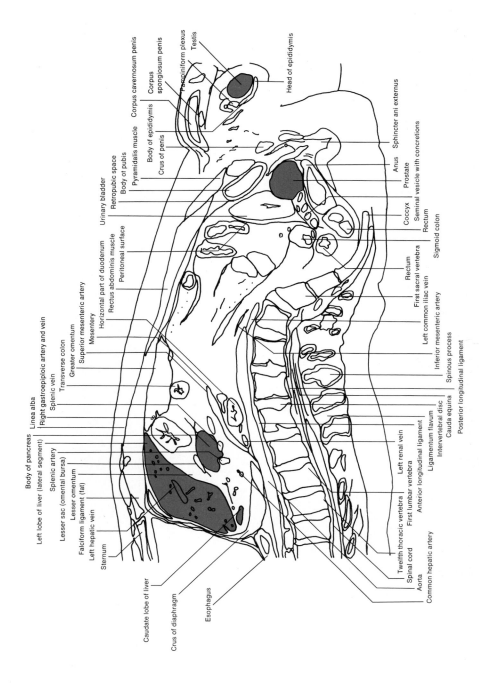

Body of pancreas
Left lobe of liver (lateral segment)
Splenic artery
Lesser omentum
Falciform ligament (fat)
Left hepatic vein
Sternum

Caudate lobe of liver

Crus of diaphragm

Esophagus

Linea alba
Right gastroepiploic artery and vein
Splenic vein
Transverse colon
Greater omentum
Superior mesenteric artery
Mesentery
Horizontal part of duodenum
Rectus abdominis muscle
Peritoneal surface

Urinary bladder
Retropubic space
Body of pubis
Pyramidalis muscle
Crus of penis
Body of epididymis
Corpus cavernosum penis
Corpus spongiosum penis
Pampiniform plexus
Testis

Head of epididymis

Sphincter ani externus
Anus
Prostate
Seminal vesicle with concretions
Rectum
Sigmoid colon

Coccyx

First sacral vertebra
Left common iliac vein
Inferior mesenteric artery
Spinous process
Posterior longitudinal ligament

Twelfth thoracic vertebra
First lumbar vertebra
Anterior longitudinal ligament
Left renal vein
Ligamentum flavum
Intervertebral disc
Cauda equina

Spinal cord
Aorta
Common hepatic artery

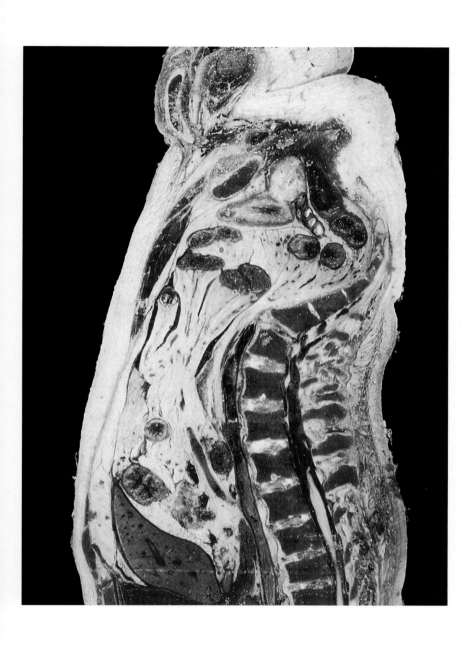

Parasagittal **Abdomen and Pelvis—Male**

Plate 92

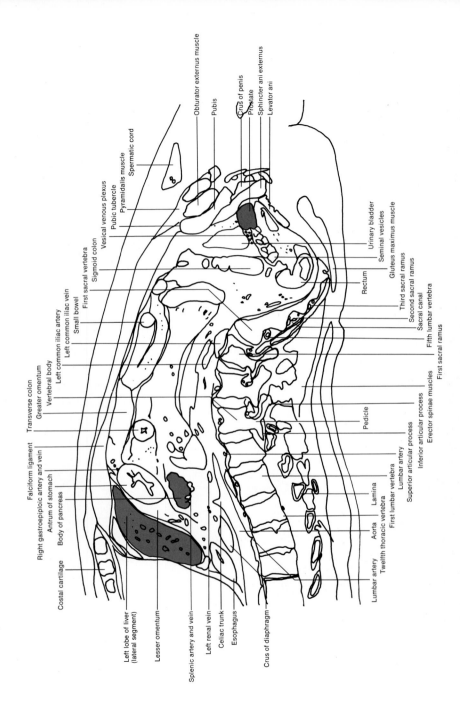

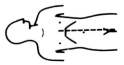

Obturator externus muscle
Pubis
Crus of penis
Prostate
Sphincter ani externus
Levator ani

Spermatic cord
Pyramidalis muscle
Pubic tubercle
Vesical venous plexus

Sigmoid colon
First sacral vertebra
Small bowel
Left common iliac vein
Left common iliac artery

Vertebral body
Greater omentum
Transverse colon

Falciform ligament
Right gastroepiploic artery and vein
Antrum of stomach
Body of pancreas

Costal cartilage

Left lobe of liver (lateral segment)
Lesser omentum
Splenic artery and vein
Left renal vein
Celiac trunk
Esophagus
Crus of diaphragm

Lumbar artery
Twelfth thoracic vertebra
Aorta
First lumbar vertebra
Lumbar artery
Superior articular process
Inferior articular process
Erector spinae muscles

Lamina

Pedicle

First sacral ramus
Fifth lumbar vertebra
Sacral canal
Second sacral ramus
Third sacral ramus

Rectum

Urinary bladder
Seminal vesicles
Gluteus maximus muscle

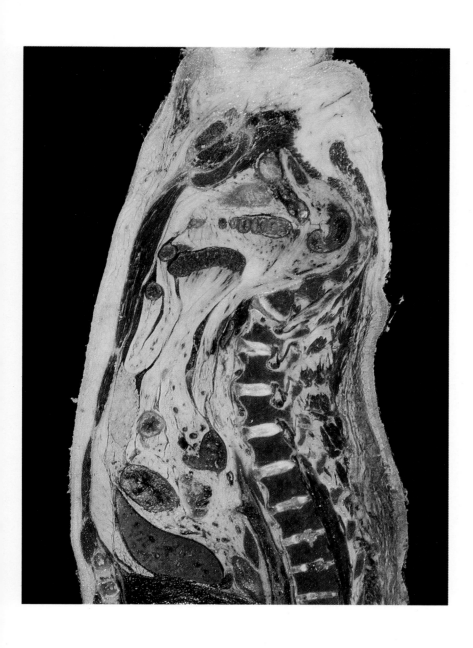

Parasagittal **Abdomen and Pelvis—Male**

Plate 93

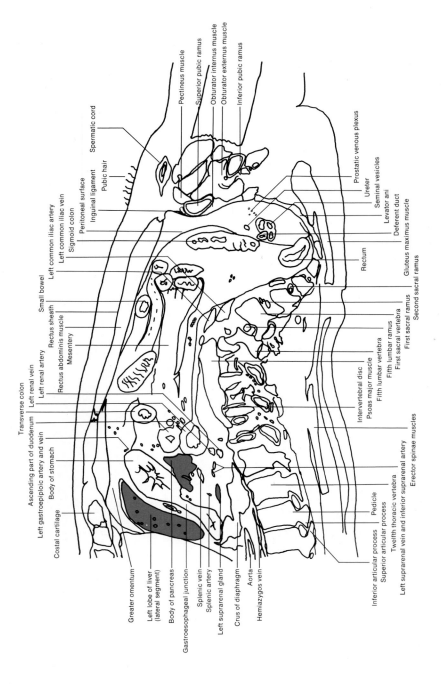

Pectineus muscle
Superior pubic ramus
Obturator internus muscle
Obturator externus muscle
Inferior pubic ramus

Spermatic cord

Prostatic venous plexus
Ureter
Seminal vesicles
Levator ani
Deferent duct
Gluteus maximus muscle

Rectum

Peritoneal surface
Inguinal ligament
Pubic hair

Left common iliac artery
Left common iliac vein
Sigmoid colon

Small bowel

Left renal artery
Rectus sheath
Rectus abdominis muscle
Mesentery

Transverse colon
Ascending part of duodenum
Left gastroepiploic artery and vein
Body of stomach

Costal cartilage

Greater omentum
Left lobe of liver
(lateral segment)
Body of pancreas
Gastroesophageal junction
Splenic vein
Splenic artery
Left suprarenal gland
Crus of diaphragm
Aorta
Hemiazygos vein

Inferior articular process
Superior articular process
Twelfth thoracic vertebra
Left suprarenal vein and inferior suprarenal artery
Erector spinae muscles

Pedicle

Intervertebral disc
Psoas major muscle
Fifth lumbar vertebra
First lumbar vertebra
First sacral ramus
Second sacral ramus

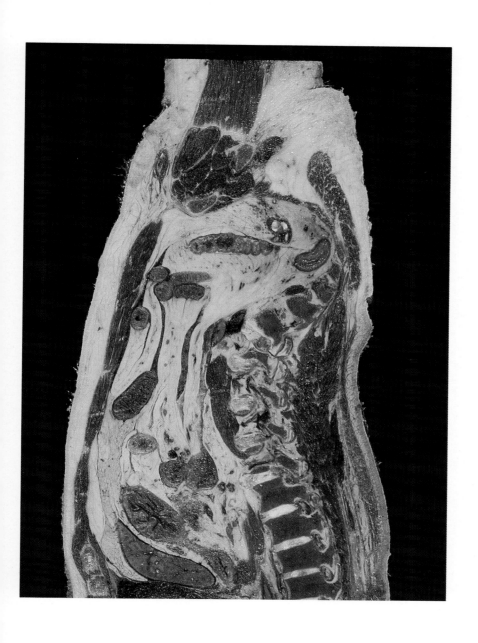

Plate 94

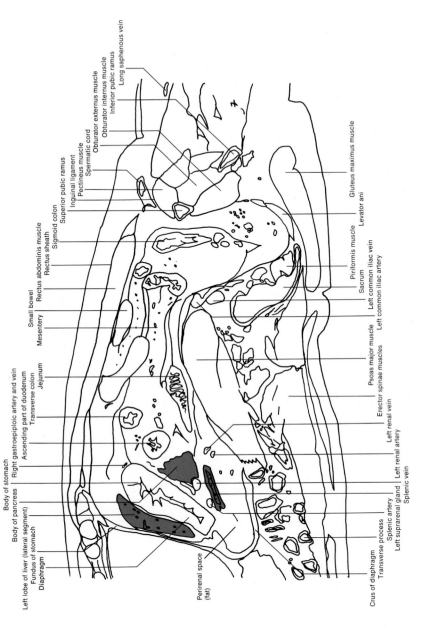

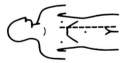

Body of stomach
Body of pancreas
Left lobe of liver (lateral segment)
Fundus of stomach
Diaphragm

Right gastroepiploic artery and vein
Ascending part of duodenum
Transverse colon
Jejunum

Small bowel
Mesentery
Rectus abdominis muscle
Rectus sheath
Sigmoid colon
Superior pubic ramus
Inguinal ligament
Pectineus muscle
Spermatic cord
Obturator externus muscle
Obturator internus muscle
Inferior pubic ramus
Long saphenous vein

Perirenal space
(fat)

Crus of diaphragm
Transverse process
Splenic artery
Left suprarenal gland
Splenic vein
Left renal artery
Left renal vein

Psoas major muscle
Erector spinae muscles
Left common iliac artery
Left common iliac vein
Sacrum
Piriformis muscle
Levator ani
Gluteus maximus muscle

Parasagittal **Abdomen and Pelvis—Male**

Plate 95

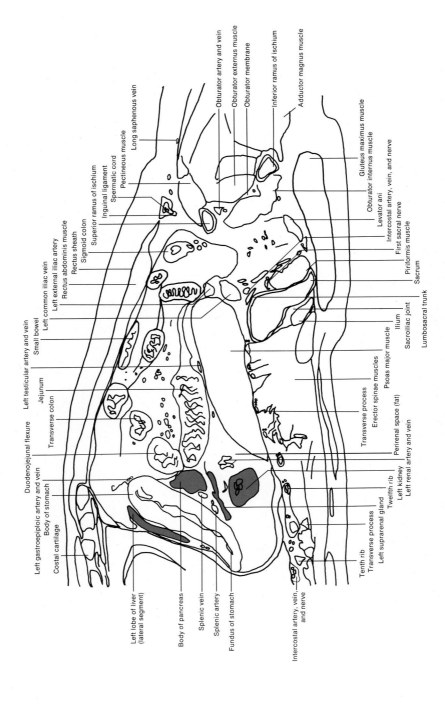

Left lobe of liver (lateral segment)

Body of pancreas

Splenic vein

Splenic artery

Fundus of stomach

Intercostal artery, vein, and nerve

Tenth rib

Transverse process

Left suprarenal gland

Twelfth rib

Left kidney

Left renal artery and vein

Transverse process

Erector spinae muscles

Perirenal space (fat)

Transverse process

Psoas major muscle

Ilium

Sacroiliac joint

Lumbosacral trunk

Sacrum

Piriformis muscle

First sacral nerve

Intercostal artery, vein, and nerve

Levator ani

Obturator internus muscle

Gluteus maximus muscle

Adductor magnus muscle

Inferior ramus of ischium

Obturator membrane

Obturator externus muscle

Obturator artery and vein

Long saphenous vein

Pectineous muscle

Spermatic cord

Inguinal ligament

Superior ramus of ischium

Sigmoid colon

Rectus sheath

Rectus abdominis muscle

Left external iliac artery

Left common iliac vein

Small bowel

Left testicular artery and vein

Jejunum

Transverse colon

Duodenojejunal flexure

Left gastroepiploic artery and vein

Body of stomach

Costal cartilage

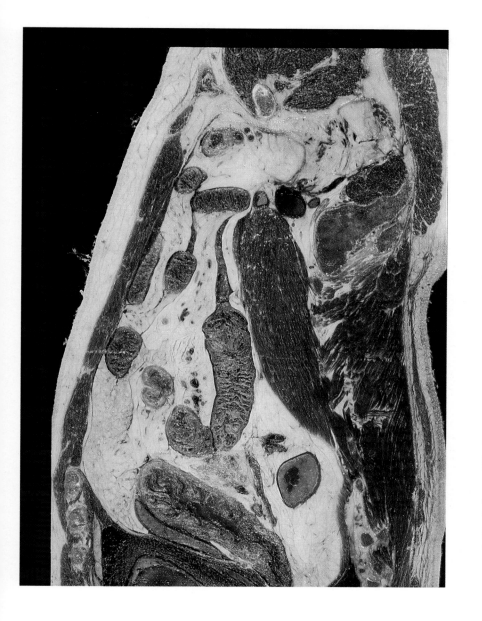

Plate 96

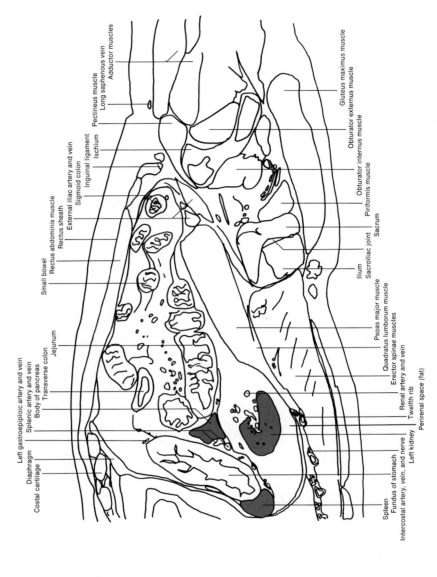

Pectineus muscle
Long saphenous vein
Adductor muscles

Gluteus maximus muscle

Obturator externus muscle

Obturator internus muscle

Piriformis muscle

Sacrum

Sacroiliac joint

Ilium

Psoas major muscle

Quadratus lumborum muscle

Erector spinae muscles

Renal artery and vein

Twelfth rib

Perirenal space (fat)

Inguinal ligament
Ischium

External iliac artery and vein
Sigmoid colon

Rectus abdominis muscle
Rectus sheath

Small bowel

Left gastroepiploic artery and vein
Splenic artery and vein
Body of pancreas
Transverse colon
Jejunum

Diaphragm
Costal cartilage

Spleen
Fundus of stomach
Intercostal artery, vein, and nerve
Left kidney

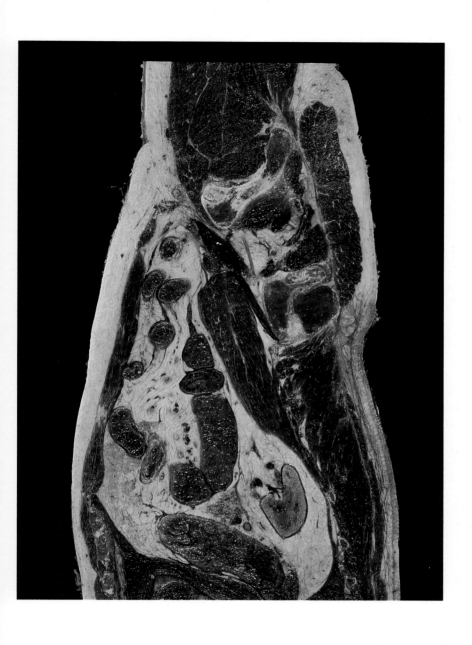

Parasagittal **Abdomen and Pelvis—Male**

Plate 97

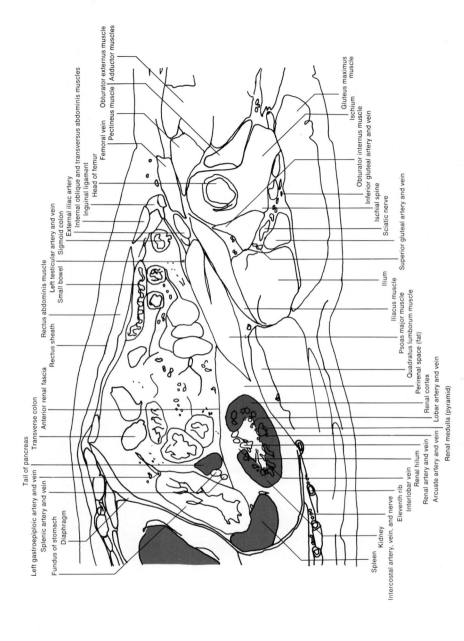

Left gastroepiploic artery and vein
Tail of pancreas
Splenic artery and vein
Fundus of stomach
Diaphragm

Transverse colon
Anterior renal fascia
Rectus sheath
Rectus abdominis muscle
Left testicular artery and vein
Small bowel
Sigmoid colon
Internal oblique and transversus abdominis muscles
Inguinal ligament
Head of femur
External iliac artery
Femoral vein
Pectineus muscle
Obturator externus muscle
Adductor muscles

Gluteus maximus muscle
Ischium
Obturator internus muscle
Inferior gluteal artery and vein
Ischial spine
Sciatic nerve
Superior gluteal artery and vein
Ilium
Iliacus muscle
Psoas major muscle
Quadratus lumborum muscle
Perirenal space (fat)
Renal cortex
Lobar artery and vein
Renal medulla (pyramid)
Arcuate artery and vein
Renal artery and vein
Renal hilum
Interlobar vein
Eleventh rib
Intercostal artery, vein, and nerve
Kidney
Spleen

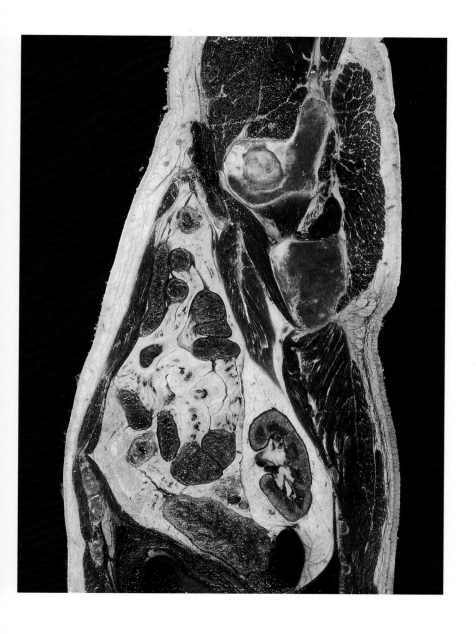

Parasagittal **Abdomen and Pelvis—Male**

Plate 98

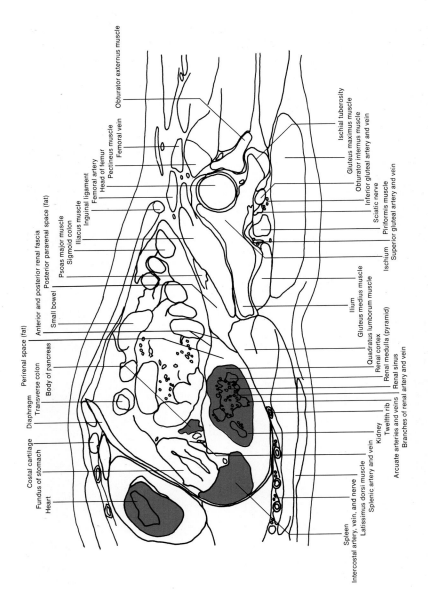

Obturator externus muscle

Ischial tuberosity
Gluteus maximus muscle
Obturator internus muscle
Inferior gluteal artery and vein
Sciatic nerve
Piriformis muscle
Superior gluteal artery and vein
Ischium

Ilium
Gluteus medius muscle
Quadratus lumborum muscle
Renal cortex
Renal medulla (pyramid)
Renal sinus
Arcuate arteries and veins
Branches of renal artery and vein

Femoral vein
Pectineus muscle
Head of femur
Femoral artery
Inguinal ligament
Iliacus muscle
Sigmoid colon
Psoas major muscle

Anterior and posterior renal fascia
Posterior pararenal space (fat)
Small bowel

Perirenal space (fat)
Diaphragm
Transverse colon
Body of pancreas

Costal cartilage
Fundus of stomach
Heart

Spleen
Intercostal artery, vein, and nerve
Latissimus dorsi muscle
Splenic artery and vein
Kidney
Twelfth rib

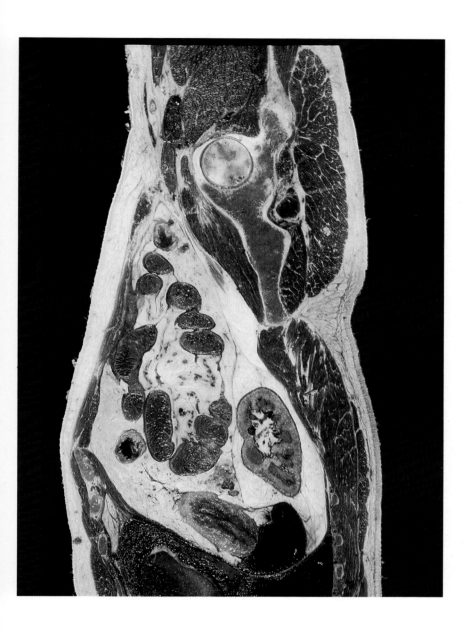

Parasagittal **Abdomen and Pelvis—Male**

Plate 99

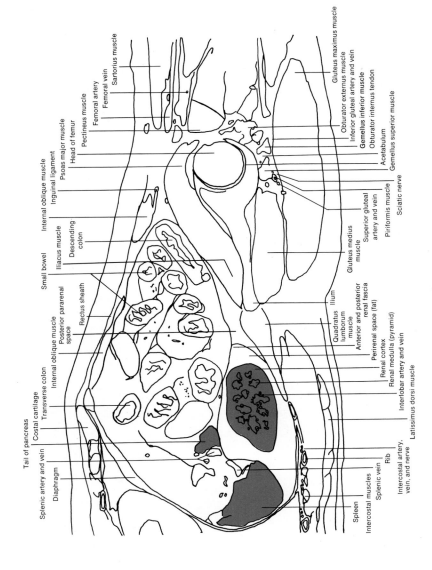
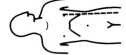

Tail of pancreas

Splenic artery and vein

Diaphragm

Costal cartilage

Transverse colon

Internal oblique muscle

Small bowel

Internal oblique muscle

Inguinal ligament

Psoas major muscle

Head of femur

Pectineus muscle

Femoral artery

Femoral vein

Sartorius muscle

Gluteus maximus muscle

Obturator externus muscle

Inferior gluteal artery and vein

Gemellus inferior muscle

Obturator internus tendon

Acetabulum

Gemellus superior muscle

Iliacus muscle

Descending colon

Posterior pararenal space

Rectus sheath

Superior gluteal artery and vein

Piriformis muscle

Sciatic nerve

Gluteus medius muscle

Ilium

Quadratus lumborum muscle

Anterior and posterior renal fascia

Perirenal space (fat)

Renal cortex

Renal medulla (pyramid)

Interlobar artery and vein

Latissimus dorsi muscle

Spleen

Intercostal muscles

Splenic vein

Rib

Intercostal artery, vein, and nerve

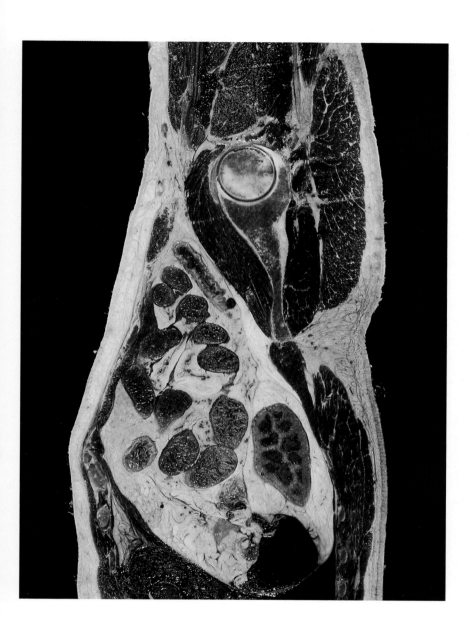

Parasagittal **Abdomen and Pelvis—Male**

Plate 100

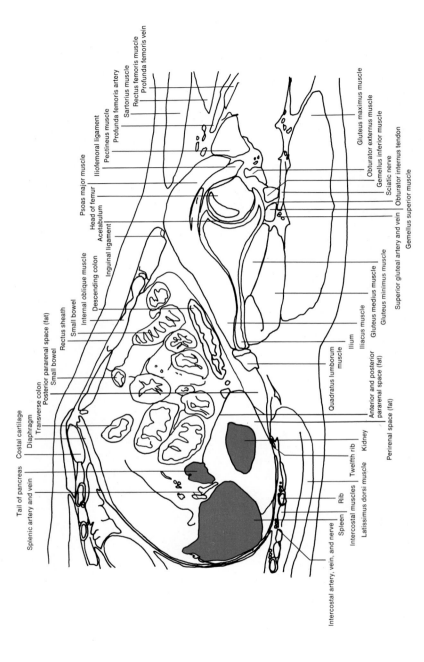

Profunda femoris vein
Profunda femoris artery
Rectus femoris muscle
Sartorius muscle
Pectineus muscle
Iliofemoral ligament

Gluteus maximus muscle
Obturator externus muscle
Gemellus inferior muscle
Sciatic nerve
Obturator internus tendon
Gemellus superior muscle

Psoas major muscle
Head of femur
Acetabulum
Inguinal ligament

Superior gluteal artery and vein

Internal oblique muscle
Descending colon
Small bowel
Rectus sheath
Small bowel
Posterior pararenal space (fat)

Ilium
Iliacus muscle
Gluteus medius muscle
Gluteus minimus muscle

Tail of pancreas
Splenic artery and vein
Costal cartilage
Diaphragm
Transverse colon

Quadratus lumborum muscle
Anterior and posterior pararenal space (fat)
Perirenal space (fat)

Kidney
Twelfth rib
Rib
Spleen
Intercostal muscles
Latissimus dorsi muscle
Intercostal artery, vein, and nerve

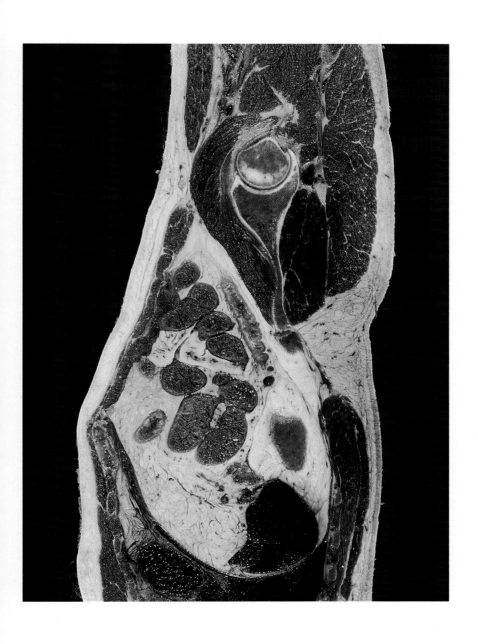

Parasagittal **Abdomen and Pelvis—Male**

Plate 101

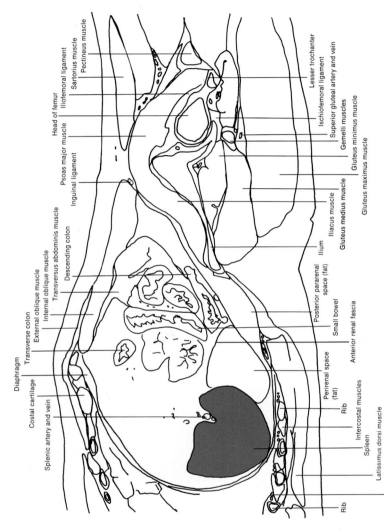

Costal cartilage

Diaphragm

Splenic artery and vein

Transverse colon

External oblique muscle

Internal oblique muscle

Transversus abdominis muscle

Descending colon

Inguinal ligament

Psoas major muscle

Head of femur

Iliofemoral ligament

Sartorius muscle

Pectineus muscle

Lesser trochanter

Ischiofemoral ligament

Superior gluteal artery and vein

Gemelli muscles

Gluteus minimus muscle

Gluteus maximus muscle

Gluteus medius muscle

Iliacus muscle

Ilium

Posterior pararenal space (fat)

Anterior renal fascia

Small bowel

Perrirenal space (fat)

Rib

Intercostal muscles

Spleen

Latissimus dorsi muscle

Rib

Intercostal artery, vein, and nerve

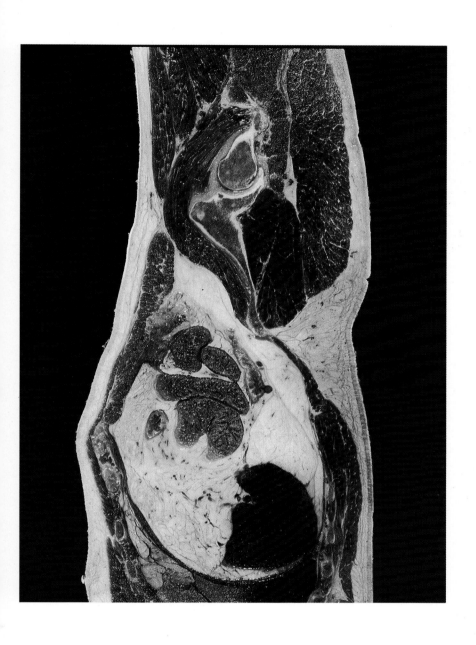

Parasagittal **Abdomen and Pelvis—Male**

Plate 102

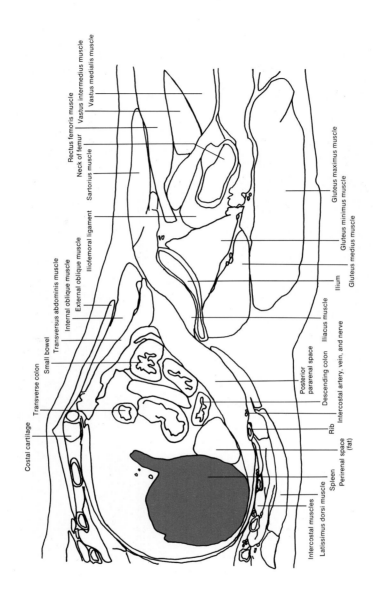

Costal cartilage

Transverse colon

Small bowel

Transversus abdominis muscle

Internal oblique muscle

External oblique muscle

Iliofemoral ligament

Sartorius muscle

Rectus femoris muscle

Neck of femur

Vastus intermedius muscle

Vastus medialis muscle

Gluteus maximus muscle

Gluteus minimus muscle

Gluteus medius muscle

Ilium

Iliacus muscle

Descending colon

Posterior
pararenal space

Intercostal artery, vein, and nerve

Rib

Perirenal space
(fat)

Spleen

Latissimus dorsi muscle

Intercostal muscles

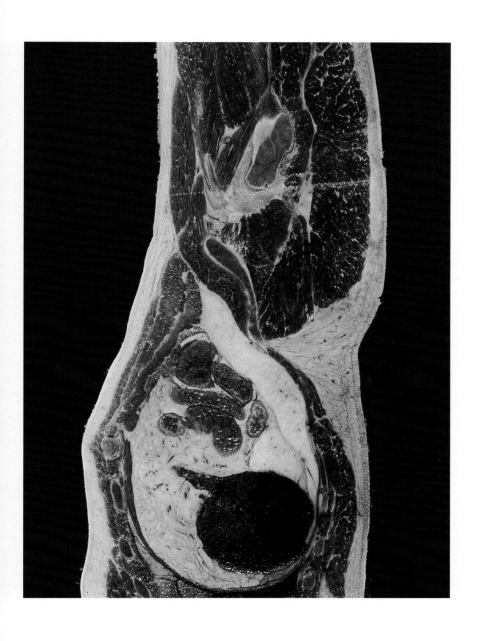

Plate 103

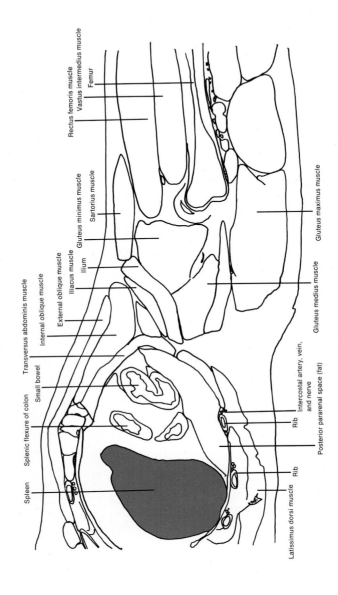

Rectus femoris muscle
Vastus intermedius muscle
Femur

Gluteus minimus muscle
Sartorius muscle

Gluteus maximus muscle

Ilium

Gluteus medius muscle

Transversus abdominis muscle

Internal oblique muscle

External oblique muscle

Iliacus muscle

Intercostal artery, vein, and nerve

Small bowel

Posterior pararenal space (fat)

Splenic flexure of colon

Rib

Spleen

Rib

Latissimus dorsi muscle

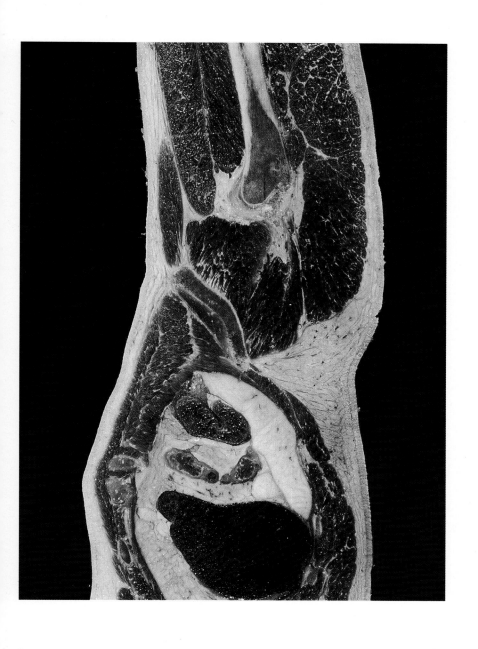

Parasagittal **Abdomen and Pelvis—Male**

Plate 104

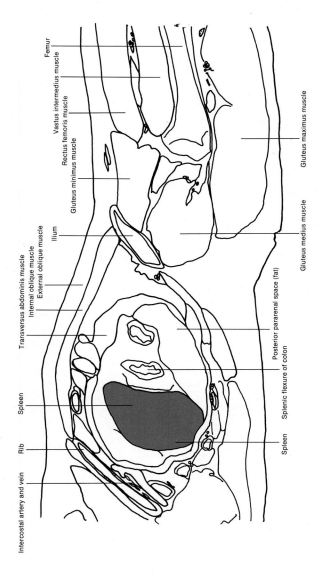

Intercostal artery and vein

Rib

Spleen

Transversus abdominis muscle
Internal oblique muscle
External oblique muscle

Ilium

Gluteus minimus muscle

Rectus femoris muscle

Vastus intermedius muscle

Femur

Gluteus maximus muscle

Gluteus medius muscle

Posterior pararenal space (fat)

Splenic flexure of colon

Spleen

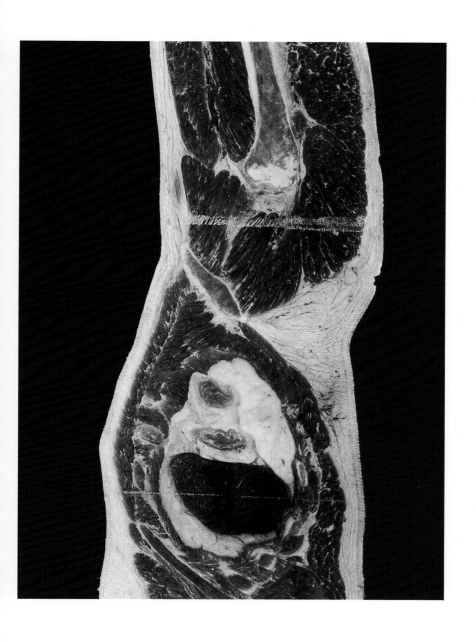

Plate 105

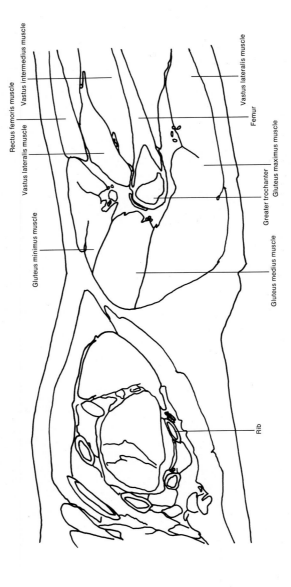

Rectus femoris muscle
Vastus intermedius muscle
Vastus lateralis muscle
Gluteus minimus muscle
Gluteus medius muscle
Greater trochanter
Gluteus maximus muscle
Femur
Vastus lateralis muscle
Rib

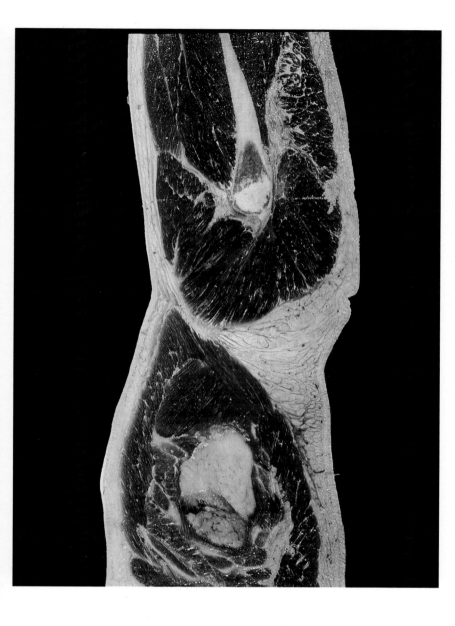

Parasagittal **Abdomen and Pelvis—Male**

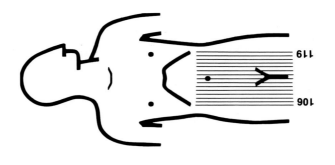

PARASAGITTAL **Pelvis—Female** *Plates 106–119*

Plate 106

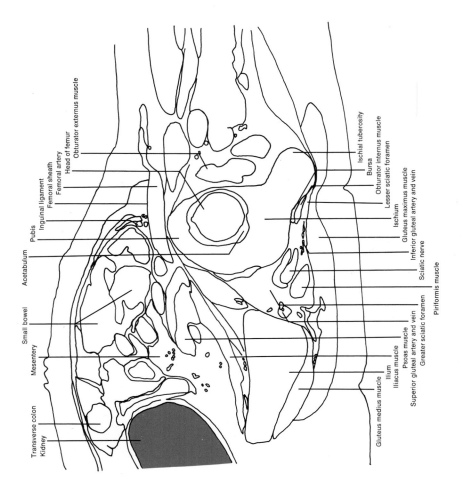

Transverse colon
Kidney

Mesentery

Small bowel

Acetabulum

Pubis

Inguinal ligament
Femoral sheath
Femoral artery
Head of femur
Obturator externus muscle

Ischial tuberosity

Bursa
Obturator internus muscle
Lesser sciatic foramen

Ischium
Gluteus maximus muscle

Inferior gluteal artery and vein

Sciatic nerve

Piriformis muscle

Gluteus medius muscle
Ilium
Iliacus muscle
Psoas muscle
Superior gluteal artery and vein
Greater sciatic foramen

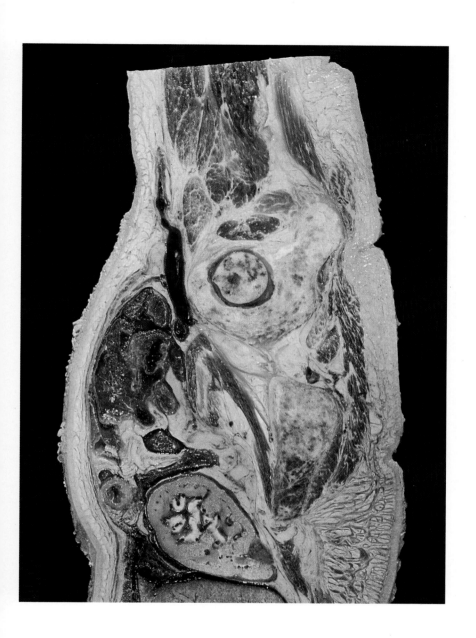

Parasagittal **Pelvis—Female**

Plate 107

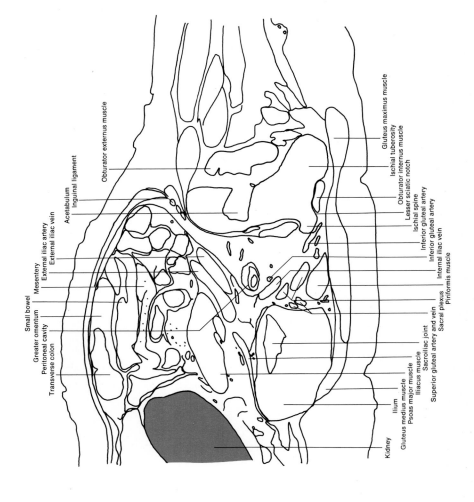

Obturator externus muscle

Acetabulum
Inguinal ligament

External iliac artery
External iliac vein

Mesentery
Small bowel

Greater omentum
Peritoneal cavity
Transverse colon

Kidney

Ilium
Gluteus medius muscle
Psoas major muscle
Iliacus muscle
Sacroiliac joint
Superior gluteal artery and vein
Sacral plexus

Gluteus maximus muscle
Ischial tuberosity
Obturator internus muscle
Lesser sciatic notch
Ischial spine
Inferior gluteal artery
Inferior gluteal vein
Internal iliac vein
Piriformis muscle

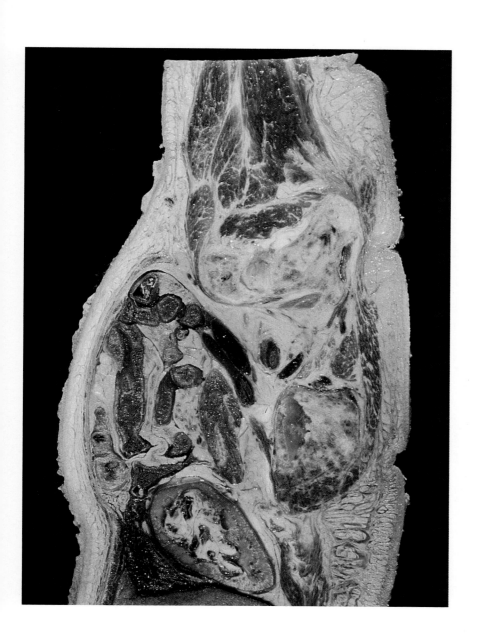

Parasagittal **Pelvis—Female**

Plate 108

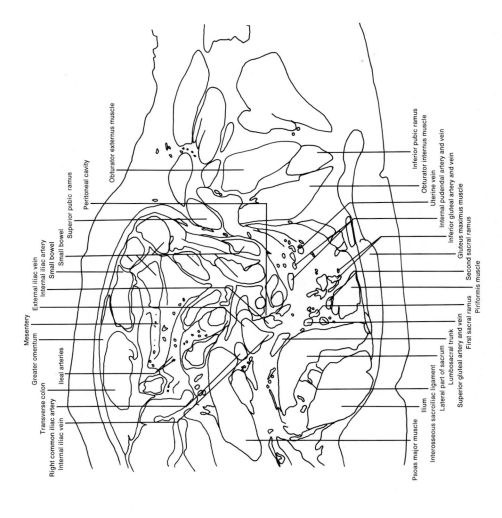

Obturator externus muscle

Peritoneal cavity

Superior pubic ramus

Small bowel

Internal iliac artery

External iliac vein

Mesentery

Greater omentum

Ileal arteries

Transverse colon

Right common iliac artery

Internal iliac vein

Psoas major muscle

Interosseous sacroiliac ligament

Ilium

Lateral part of sacrum

Lumbosacral trunk

Superior gluteal artery and vein

First sacral ramus

Piriformis muscle

Second sacral ramus

Gluteus maximus muscle

Inferior gluteal artery and vein

Internal pudendal artery and vein

Uterine vein

Obturator internus muscle

Inferior pubic ramus

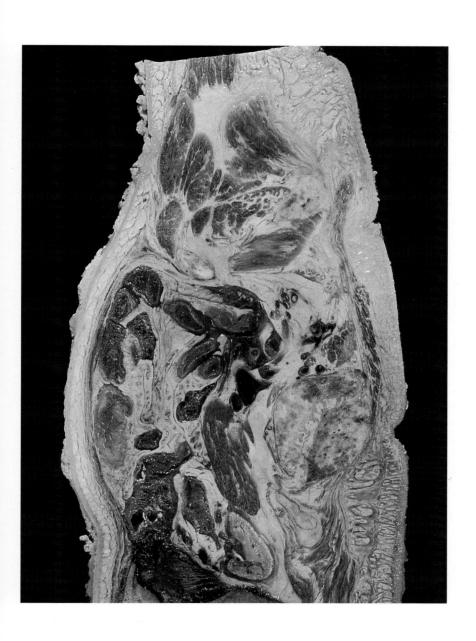

Parasagittal **Pelvis—Female**

Plate 109

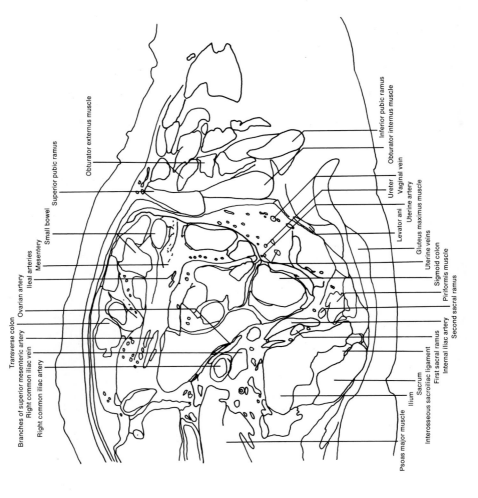

Transverse colon
Branches of superior mesenteric artery
Right common iliac vein
Right common iliac artery

Ovarian artery
Ileal arteries
Mesentery
Small bowel
Superior pubic ramus

Obturator externus muscle

Inferior pubic ramus
Obturator internus muscle

Ureter
Vaginal vein
Uterine artery
Levator ani
Uterine veins
Gluteus maximus muscle
Sigmoid colon
Piriformis muscle
Second sacral ramus

Psoas major muscle
Ilium
Sacrum
Interosseous sacroiliac ligament
First sacral ramus
Internal iliac artery

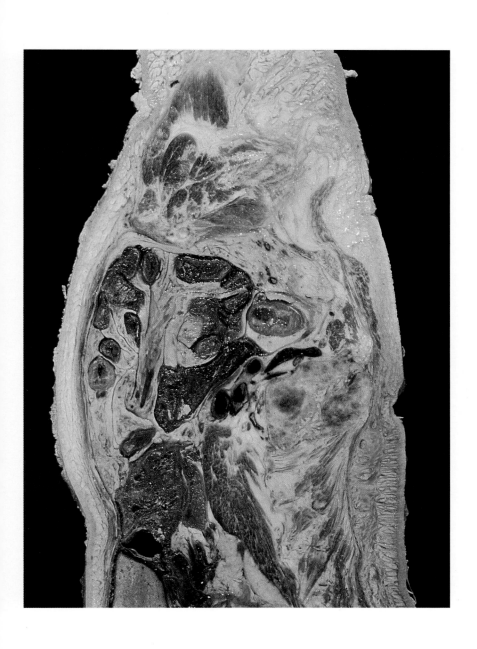

Parasagittal **Pelvis—Female**

Plate 110

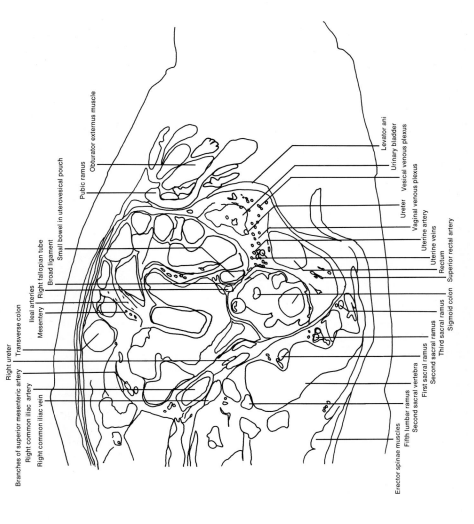

Right ureter
Transverse colon
Branches of superior mesenteric artery
Right common iliac artery
Right common iliac vein

Ileal arteries
Mesentery
Right fallopian tube
Broad ligament
Small bowel in uterovesical pouch
Pubic ramus
Obturator externus muscle

Levator ani
Urinary bladder
Vesical venous plexus
Ureter
Vaginal venous plexus
Uterine artery
Uterine veins
Rectum
Superior rectal artery

Erector spinae muscles
Fifth lumbar ramus
Second sacral vertebra
First sacral ramus
Second sacral ramus
Third sacral ramus
Sigmoid colon

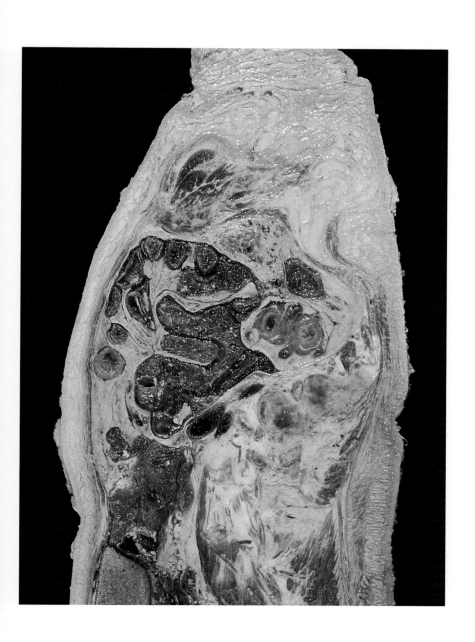

Parasagittal **Pelvis—Female**

Plate 111

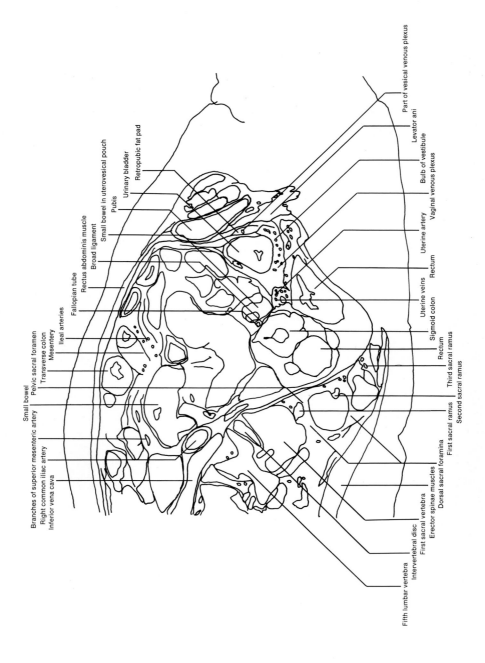

Small bowel
Branches of superior mesenteric artery
Right common iliac artery
Inferior vena cava

Pelvic sacral foramen
Transverse colon
Mesentery
Ileal arteries
Fallopian tube
Rectus abdominis muscle
Broad ligament
Small bowel in uterovesical pouch
Pubis
Urinary bladder
Retropubic fat pad

Part of vesical venous plexus
Levator ani
Bulb of vestibule
Vaginal venous plexus
Uterine artery
Rectum
Uterine veins
Sigmoid colon
Rectum
Third sacral ramus
Second sacral ramus
First sacral ramus
Dorsal sacral foramina
Erector spinae muscles
First sacral vertebra
Intervertebral disc
Fifth lumbar vertebra

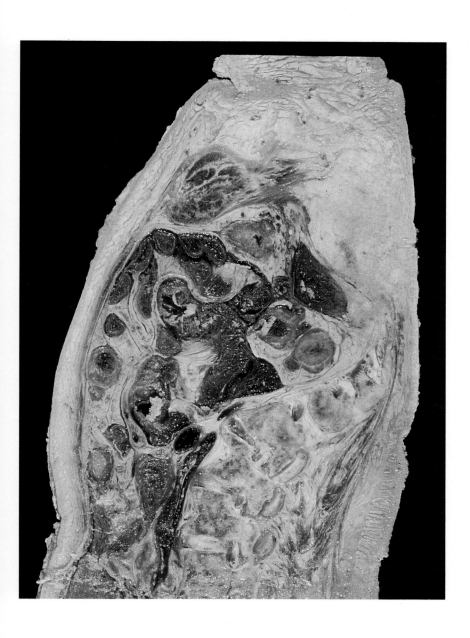

Parasagittal **Pelvis—Female**

Plate 112

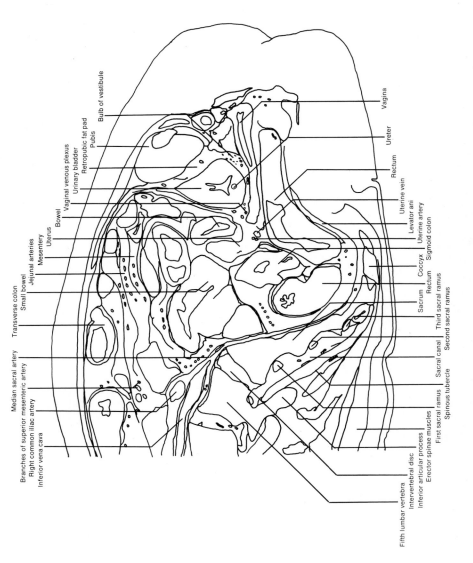

Transverse colon

Median sacral artery

Branches of superior mesenteric artery
Right common iliac artery
Inferior vena cava

Small bowel
Jejunal arteries
Mesentery
Uterus
Bowel

Vaginal venous plexus
Urinary bladder
Retropubic fat pad
Pubis
Bulb of vestibule

Vagina

Ureter

Rectum

Uterine vein
Levator ani
Uterine artery
Sigmoid colon

Sacrum
Coccyx
Rectum
Third sacral ramus

Second sacral ramus

Sacral canal

Spinous tubercle

First sacral ramus

Erector spinae muscles

Inferior articular process

Intervertebral disc

Fifth lumbar vertebra

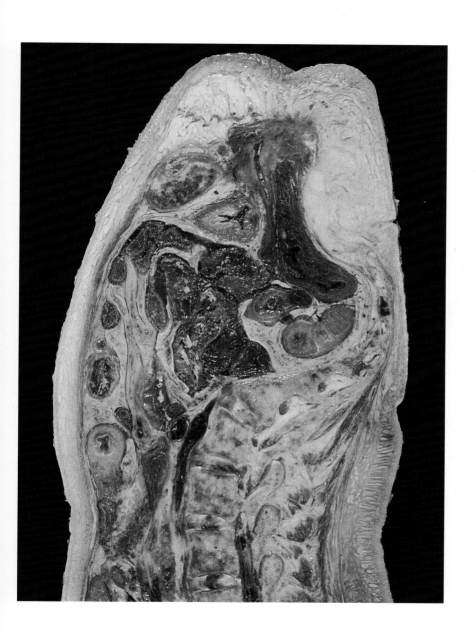

Parasagittal **Pelvis—Female**

Plate 113

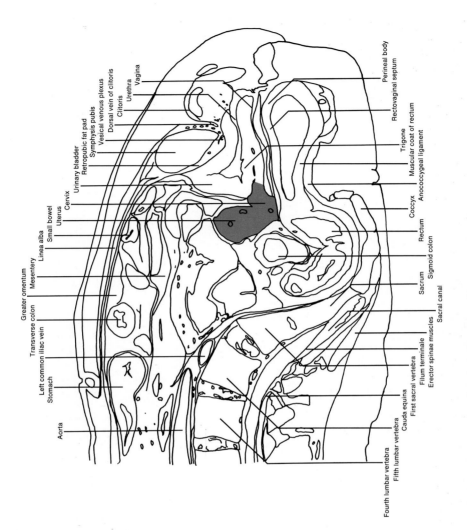

Perineal body

Rectovaginal septum

Vagina
Urethra
Clitoris
Dorsal vein of clitoris
Vesical venous plexus
Symphysis pubis
Retropubic fat pad
Urinary bladder

Trigone
Muscular coat of rectum
Anococcygeal ligament

Coccyx

Rectum

Sigmoid colon

Sacrum

Sacral canal

Erector spinae muscles
Filum terminale
First sacral vertebra
Cauda equina
Fifth lumbar vertebra
Fourth lumbar vertebra

Cervix
Uterus
Small bowel
Linea alba
Mesentery
Greater omentum
Transverse colon
Left common iliac vein
Stomach

Aorta

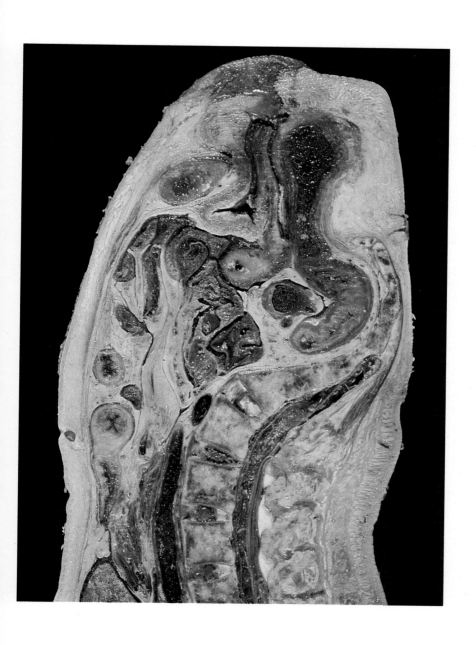

Parasagittal **Pelvis—Female**

Plate 114

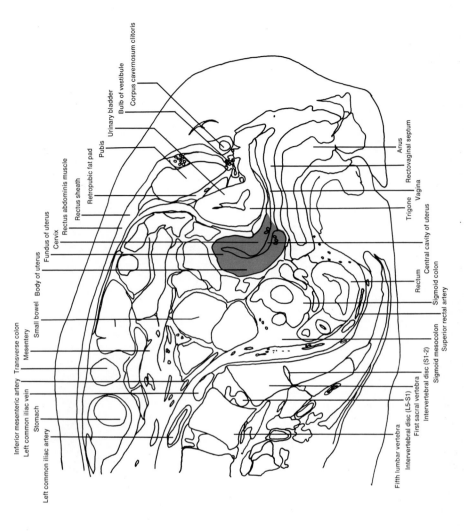

Inferior mesenteric artery
Left common iliac vein
Left common iliac artery
Stomach
Transverse colon
Mesentery
Small bowel
Body of uterus
Fundus of uterus
Cervix
Rectus abdominis muscle
Rectus sheath
Retropubic fat pad
Pubis
Urinary bladder
Bulb of vestibule
Corpus cavernosum clitoris

Fifth lumbar vertebra
Intervertebral disc (L5-S1)
First sacral vertebra
Intervertebral disc (S1-2)
Sigmoid mesocolon
Superior rectal artery
Sigmoid colon
Rectum
Central cavity of uterus
Trigone
Vagina
Rectovaginal septum
Anus

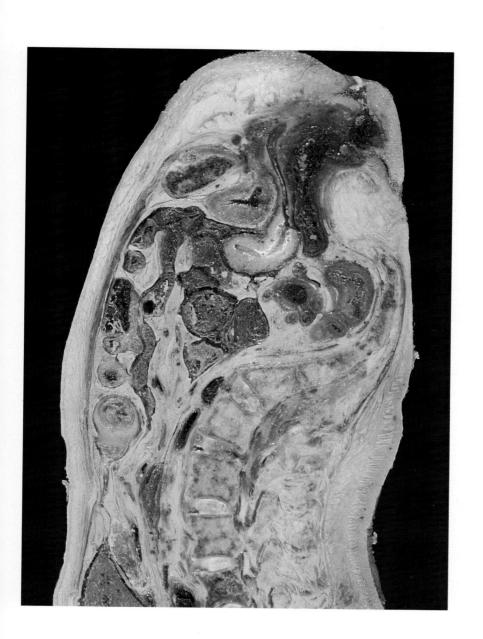

Parasagittal **Pelvis—Female**

Plate 115

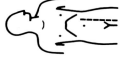

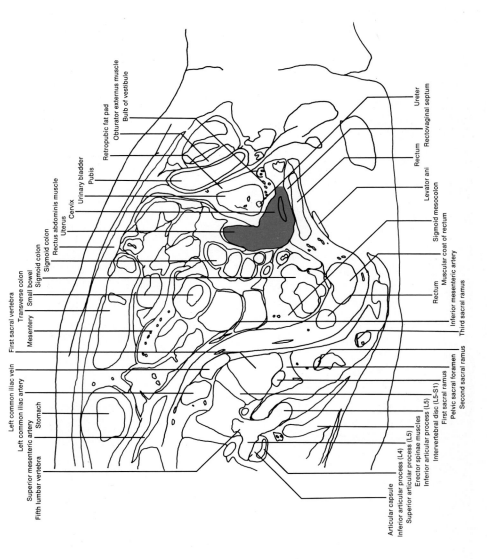

Superior mesenteric artery
Fifth lumbar vertebra
Left common iliac vein
Left common iliac artery
Stomach

First sacral vertebra
Transverse colon
Mesentery
Small bowel
Sigmoid colon
Sigmoid colon
Rectus abdominis muscle
Uterus
Cervix
Urinary bladder
Pubis
Retropubic fat pad
Obturator externus muscle
Bulb of vestibule

Ureter
Rectovaginal septum
Rectum
Levator ani
Sigmoid mesocolon
Muscular coat of rectum
Rectum
Inferior mesenteric artery
Third sacral ramus
Second sacral ramus
Pelvic sacral foramen
First sacral ramus
Intervertebral disc (L5-S1)
Inferior articular process (L5)
Erector spinae muscles
Superior articular process (L5)
Inferior articular process (L4)
Articular capsule

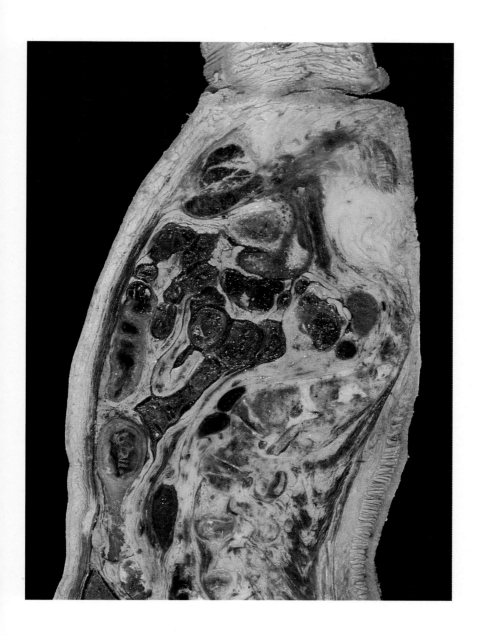

Parasagittal **Pelvis—Female**

Plate 116

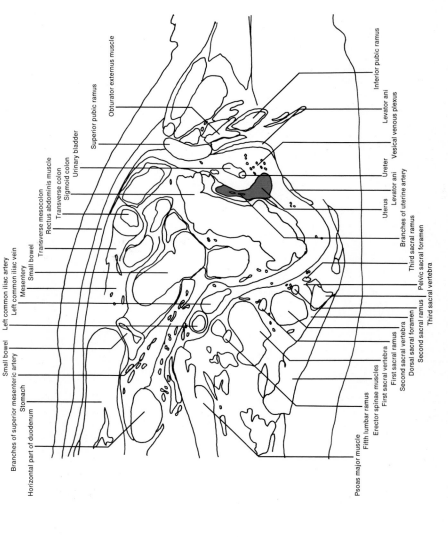

Branches of superior mesenteric artery
Small bowel
Left common iliac artery
Left common iliac vein
Stomach
Horizontal part of duodenum
Mesentery
Small bowel
Transverse mesocolon
Rectus abdominis muscle
Transverse colon
Sigmoid colon
Urinary bladder
Superior pubic ramus
Obturator externus muscle
Inferior pubic ramus
Levator ani
Vesical venous plexus
Ureter
Levator ani
Branches of uterine artery
Uterus
Third sacral ramus
Pelvic sacral foramen
Third sacral vertebra
Second sacral ramus
Dorsal sacral foramen
Second sacral vertebra
First sacral ramus
First sacral vertebra
Fifth lumbar ramus
Erector spinae muscles
Psoas major muscle

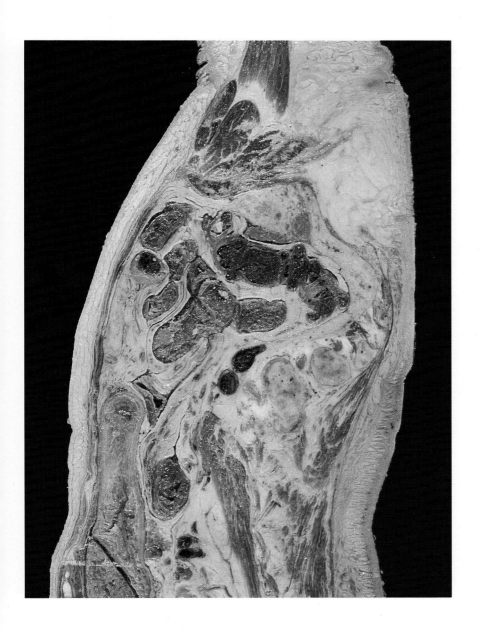

Parasagittal **Pelvis—Female**

Plate 117

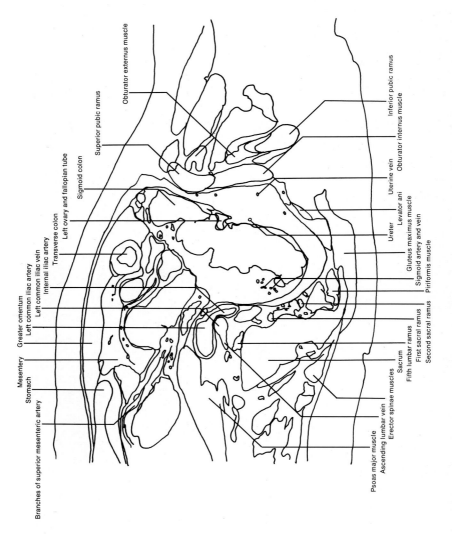

Obturator externus muscle

Superior pubic ramus

Left ovary and fallopian tube

Sigmoid colon

Transverse colon

Internal iliac artery

Left iliac vein

Left common iliac artery

Greater omentum

Mesentery

Stomach

Branches of superior mesenteric artery

Inferior pubic ramus

Obturator internus muscle

Uterine vein

Levator ani

Gluteus maximus muscle

Sigmoid artery and vein

Piriformis muscle

Ureter

Psoas major muscle

Ascending lumbar vein

Erector spinae muscles

Sacrum

Fifth lumbar ramus

First sacral ramus

Second sacral ramus

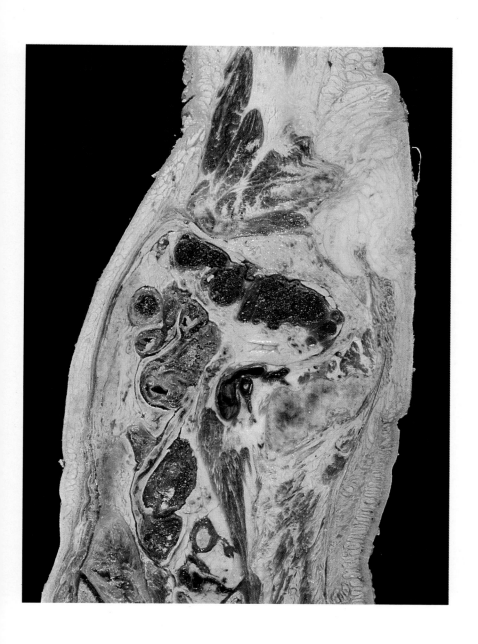

Parasagittal **Pelvis—Female**

253

Plate 118

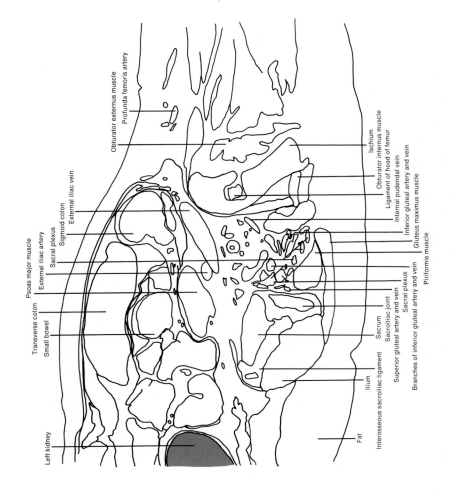

Left kidney

Transverse colon

Small bowel

Psoas major muscle

External iliac artery

Sacral plexus

Sigmoid colon

External iliac vein

Obturator externus muscle

Profunda femoris artery

Ischium

Obturator internus muscle

Ligament of head of femur

Internal pudendal vein

Inferior gluteal artery and vein

Gluteus maximus muscle

Piriformis muscle

Sacral plexus

Superior gluteal artery and vein

Sacrum

Sacroiliac joint

Branches of inferior gluteal artery and vein

Ilium

Interosseous sacroiliac ligament

Fat

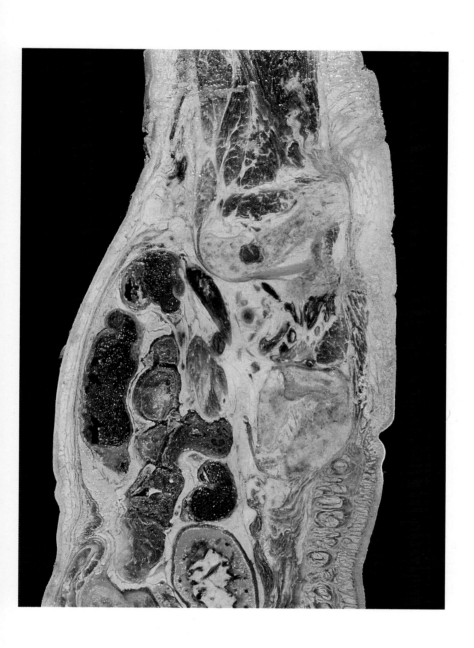

Parasagittal **Pelvis—Female**

Plate 119

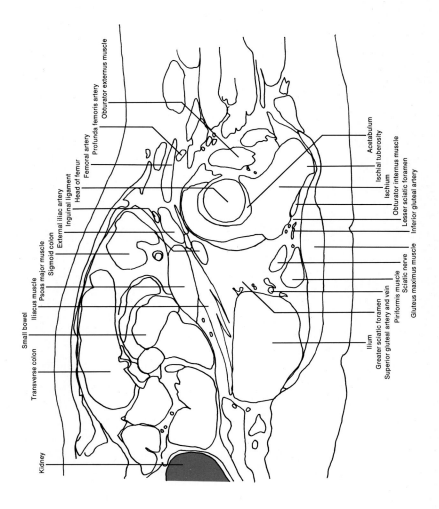

Kidney

Transverse colon

Small bowel
Iliacus muscle
Psoas major muscle
Sigmoid colon
External iliac artery
Inguinal ligament
Head of femur
Femoral artery
Profunda femoris artery
Obturator externus muscle

Acetabulum
Ischial tuberosity
Ischium
Obturator internus muscle
Lesser sciatic foramen
Inferior gluteal artery

Ilium
Greater sciatic foramen
Superior gluteal artery and vein
Piriformis muscle
Sciatic nerve
Gluteus maximus muscle

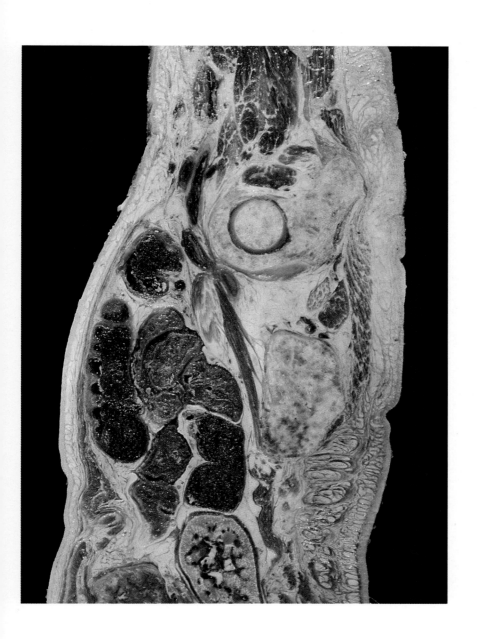

Parasagittal **Pelvis—Female**

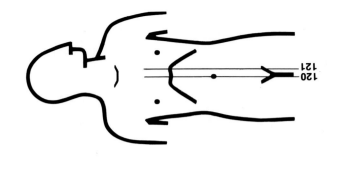

120
121

Plate 120

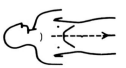

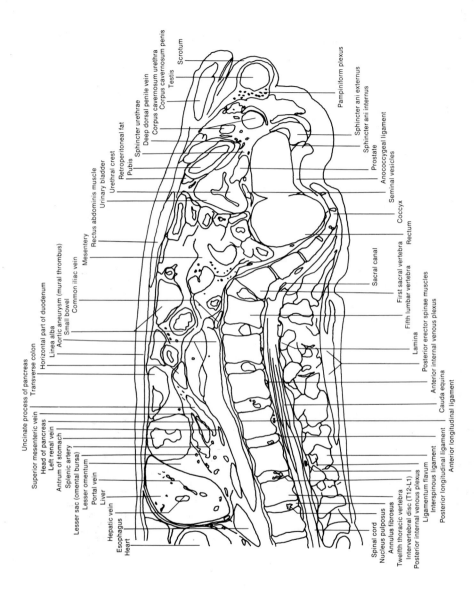

Uncinate process of pancreas
Superior mesenteric vein
Head of pancreas
Left renal vein
Splenic artery
Antrum of stomach
Lesser sac (omental bursa)
Lesser omentum
Portal vein
Liver
Hepatic vein
Esophagus
Heart

Transverse colon
Horizontal part of duodenum
Linea alba
Aortic aneurysm (mural thrombus)
Small bowel
Common iliac vein
Mesentery
Rectus abdominis muscle
Urinary bladder
Urethral crest
Retroperitoneal fat
Pubis
Sphincter urethrae
Deep dorsal penile vein
Corpus cavernosum urethra
Corpus cavernosum penis
Testis
Scrotum

Pampiniform plexus

Sphincter ani externus
Sphincter ani internus

Prostate
Anococcygeal ligament
Seminal vesicles

Coccyx

Rectum

Sacral canal

First sacral vertebra
Fifth lumbar vertebra

Lamina
Posterior erector spinae muscles
Anterior internal venous plexus

Cauda equina

Ligamentum flavum
Interspinous ligament
Posterior longitudinal ligament
Anterior longitudinal ligament

Spinal cord
Nucleus pulposus
Annulus fibrosus
Twelfth thoracic vertebra
Intervertebral disc (T12-L1)
Posterior internal venous plexus

Parasagittal **Abdominal Aortic Aneurysm**

Plate 121

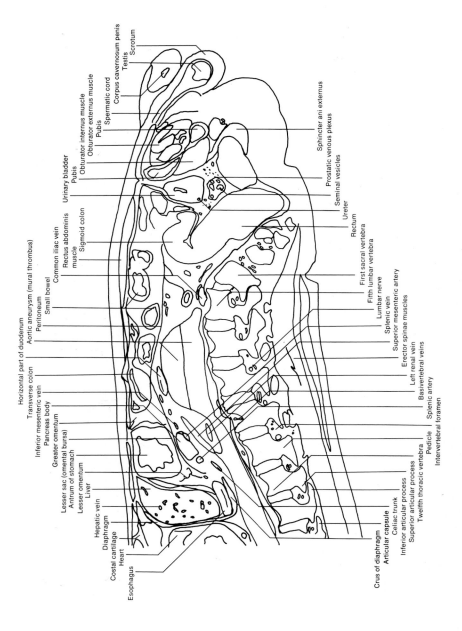

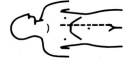

Horizontal part of duodenum
Aortic aneurysm (mural thrombus)
Transverse colon
Inferior mesenteric vein
Pancreas body
Peritoneum
Small bowel
Common iliac vein
Rectus abdominis muscle
Sigmoid colon

Greater omentum
Lesser sac (omental bursa)
Antrum of stomach
Lesser omentum
Liver
Hepatic vein
Diaphragm
Heart
Costal cartilage
Esophagus

Urinary bladder
Obturator internus muscle
Obturator externus muscle
Pubis
Pubis
Spermatic cord
Corpus cavernosum penis
Testis
Scrotum

Sphincter ani externus
Prostatic venous plexus
Seminal vesicles
Ureter
Rectum

First sacral vertebra
Fifth lumbar vertebra
Lumbar nerve
Superior mesenteric artery
Splenic vein
Erector spinae muscles
Left renal vein
Basivertebral veins
Splenic artery
Intervertebral foramen

Crus of diaphragm
Articular capsule
Celiac trunk
Inferior articular process
Superior articular process
Twelfth thoracic vertebra
Pedicle

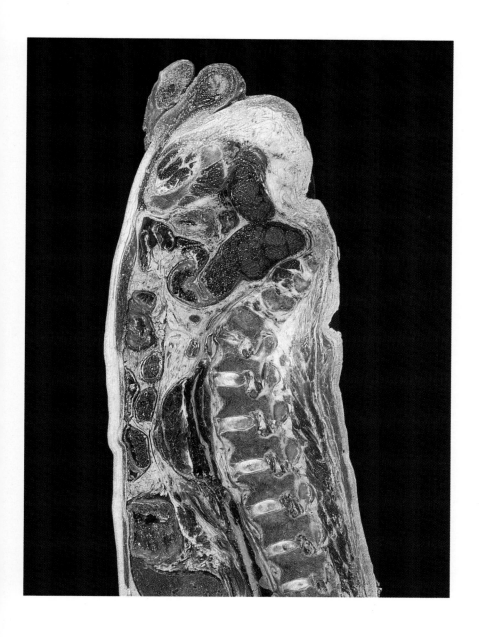

263

Part Three   CORONAL SECTIONS

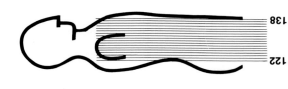

**Chest,
Abdomen,
and Pelvis**

Plates 122–138

122

138

CORONAL

Chest, Abdomen, and Pelvis   Plates 122–138

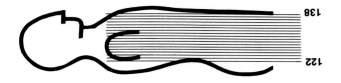

138

122

Plate 122

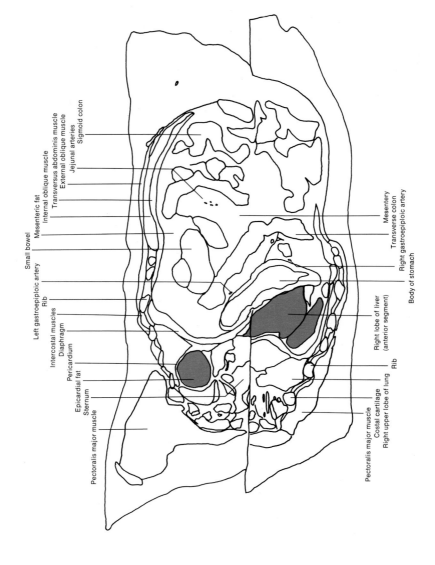

Sigmoid colon
External oblique muscle
Transversus abdominis muscle
Internal oblique muscle
Mesenteric fat

Small bowel

Left gastroepiploic artery
Rib
Intercostal muscles
Diaphragm
Pericardium
Epicardial fat
Sternum
Pectoralis major muscle

Jejunal arteries

Mesentery
Transverse colon
Right gastroepiploic artery
Body of stomach

Right lobe of liver
(anterior segment)
Rib
Costal cartilage
Right upper lobe of lung
Pectoralis major muscle

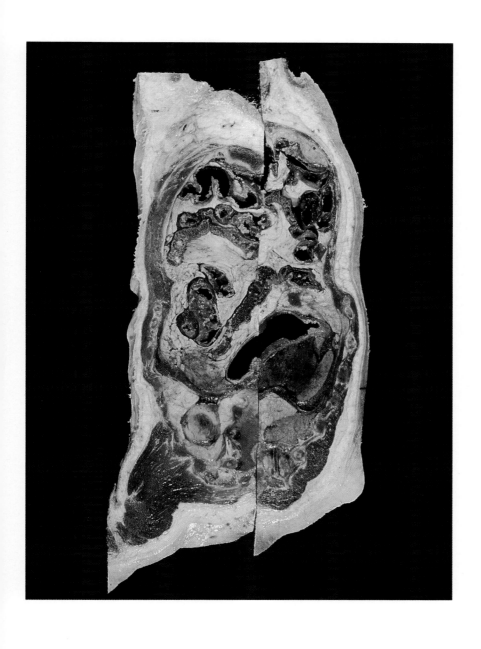

Coronal **Chest, Abdomen, and Pelvis**

Plate 123

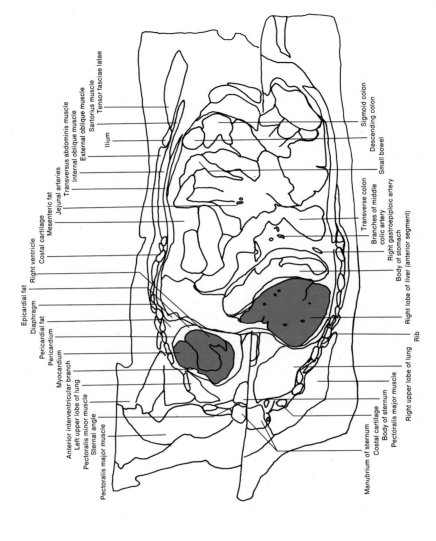

Epicardial fat
Diaphragm
Right ventricle
Costal cartilage
Mesenteric fat
Jejunal arteries
Transversus abdominis muscle
Internal oblique muscle
External oblique muscle
Sartorius muscle
Tensor fasciae latae

Pericardial fat
Pericardium
Myocardium
Anterior interventricular branch
Left upper lobe of lung
Pectoralis minor muscle
Sternal angle
Pectoralis major muscle

Ilium

Sigmoid colon
Descending colon

Small bowel

Transverse colon
Branches of middle
colic artery
Right gastroepiploic artery
Body of stomach

Right lobe of liver (anterior segment)

Rib

Right upper lobe of lung
Pectoralis major muscle
Body of sternum
Costal cartilage
Manubrium of sternum

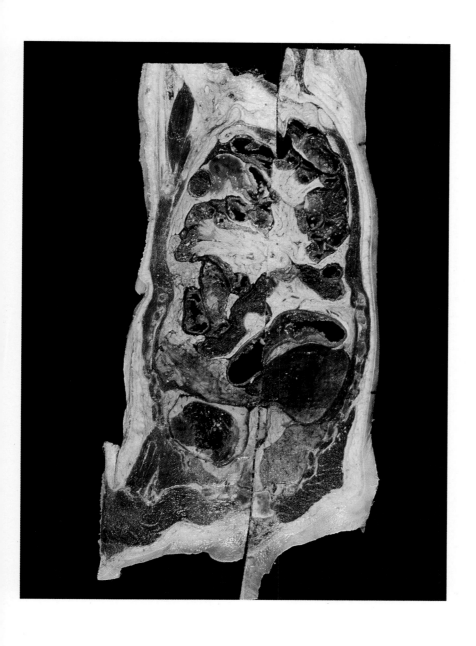

Coronal **Chest, Abdomen, and Pelvis**

Plate 124

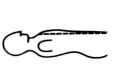

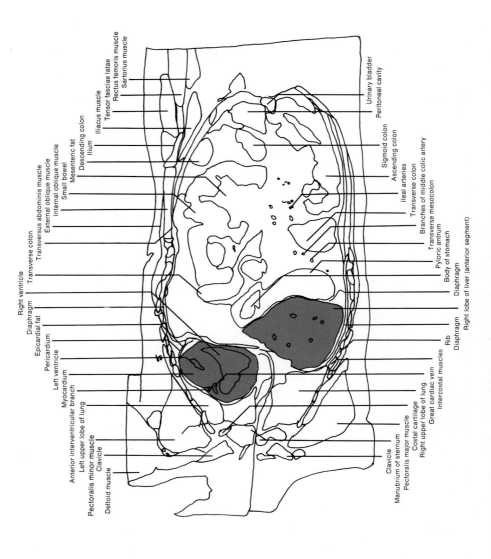

Right ventricle
Diaphragm
Epicardial fat
Pericardium
Myocardium
Left ventricle
Anterior interventricular branch
Left upper lobe of lung
Pectoralis minor muscle
Clavicle
Deltoid muscle

Transverse colon
Transversus abdominis muscle
External oblique muscle
Internal oblique muscle
Small bowel
Mesenteric fat
Descending colon
Ilium
Iliacus muscle
Tensor fasciae latae
Rectus femoris muscle
Sartorius muscle

Urinary bladder
Peritoneal cavity

Sigmoid colon
Ascending colon
Branches of middle colic artery
Ileal arteries
Transverse colon
Transverse mesocolon
Pyloric antrum
Body of stomach
Diaphragm
Right lobe of liver (anterior segment)

Diaphragm
Rib
Intercostal muscles
Great cardiac vein
Right upper lobe of lung
Costal cartilage
Pectoralis major muscle
Manubrium of sternum
Clavicle

Coronal **Chest, Abdomen, and Pelvis**

Plate 125

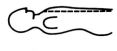

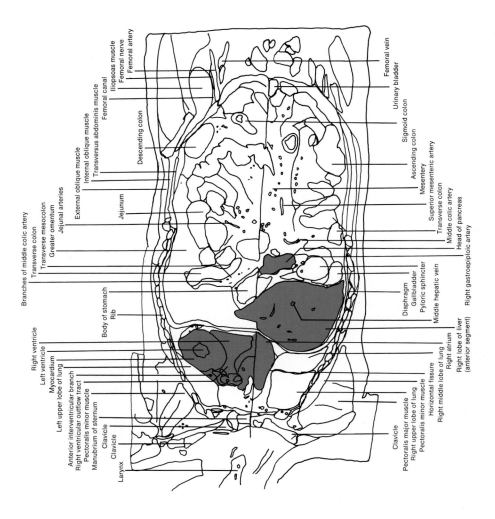

Branches of middle colic artery
Transverse colon
Transverse mesocolon
Greater omentum
Jejunal arteries

External oblique muscle

Jejunum

Right ventricle
Left ventricle
Myocardium
Anterior interventricular branch
Right ventricular outflow tract
Pectoralis minor muscle
Manubrium of sternum
Clavicle
Clavicle
Larynx

Left upper lobe of lung

Body of stomach
Rib

Descending colon

External oblique muscle
Internal oblique muscle
Transversus abdominis muscle
Femoral canal
Femoral nerve
Iliopsoas muscle
Femoral artery

Femoral vein

Urinary bladder
Sigmoid colon

Ascending colon

Mesentery
Superior mesenteric artery
Transverse colon
Middle colic artery
Head of pancreas

Right gastroepiploic artery

Diaphragm
Gallbladder
Pyloric sphincter
Middle hepatic vein

Right atrium
Right lobe of liver
(anterior segment)

Right middle lobe of lung
Horizontal fissure
Pectoralis minor muscle
Right upper lobe of lung
Pectoralis major muscle
Clavicle

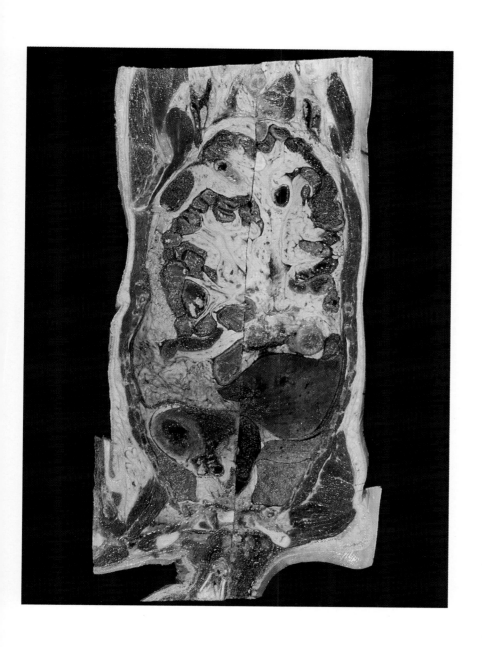

Coronal **Chest, Abdomen, and Pelvis**

Plate 126

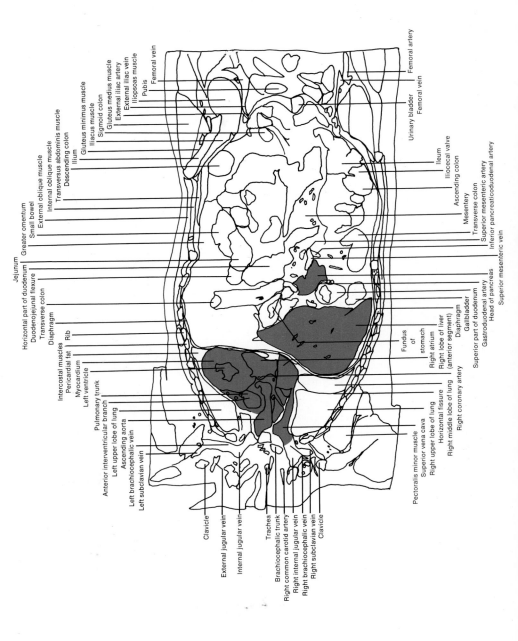

Clavicle

External jugular vein

Internal jugular vein

Trachea

Brachiocephalic trunk

Right common carotid artery

Right internal jugular vein

Right brachiocephalic vein

Right subclavian vein

Clavicle

Pectoralis minor muscle
Superior vena cava
Right upper lobe of lung
Horizontal fissure
Right middle lobe of lung
Right coronary artery

Fundus
of
stomach

Right atrium
Right lobe of liver
Right lobe of liver (anterior segment)
Diaphragm
Gallbladder
Superior part of duodenum
Gastroduodenal artery
Head of pancreas

Intercostal muscles
Pericardial fat
Myocardium
Left ventricle
Rib

Pulmonary trunk
Anterior interventricular branch
Left upper lobe of lung
Ascending aorta
Left brachiocephalic vein
Left subclavian vein

Horizontal part of duodenum
Duodenojejunal flexure
Transverse colon
Diaphragm

Jejunum
Greater omentum
Small bowel
External oblique muscle
Internal oblique muscle
Transversus abdominis muscle
Descending colon

Gluteus minimus muscle
Iliacus muscle
Gluteus medius muscle
External iliac artery
External iliac vein
Iliopsoas muscle
Ilium
Sigmoid colon
Pubis
Femoral vein

Femoral artery

Urinary bladder
Femoral vein

Ilium
Iliocecal valve
Ascending colon

Transverse colon
Mesentery
Superior mesenteric artery
Inferior pancreaticoduodenal artery

Superior mesenteric vein

Coronal **Chest, Abdomen, and Pelvis**

Plate 127

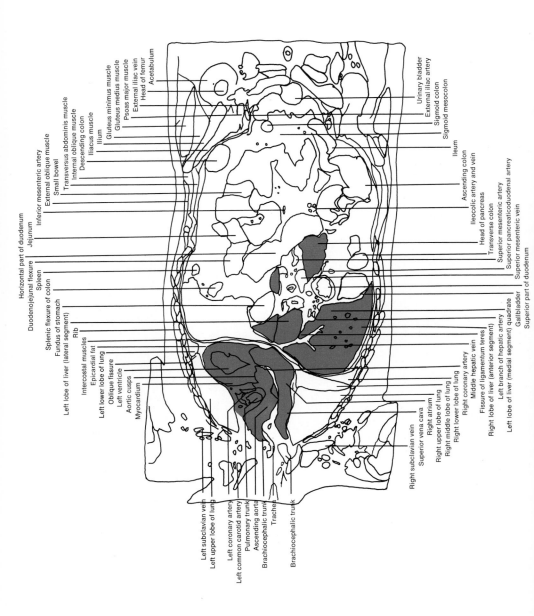

Horizontal part of duodenum
Duodenojejunal flexure
Jejunum
Splenic flexure of colon
Inferior mesenteric artery
Spleen
External oblique muscle
Fundus of stomach
Transversus abdominis muscle
Rib
Internal oblique muscle
Left lobe of liver (lateral segment)
Descending colon
Intercostal muscles
Iliacus muscle
Epicardial fat
Ilium
Left lower lobe of lung
Gluteus minimus muscle
Oblique fissure
Gluteus medius muscle
Left ventricle
Psoas major muscle
Aortic cusps
External iliac vein
Myocardium
Head of femur
Acetabulum

Urinary bladder
External iliac artery
Sigmoid colon
Sigmoid mesocolon

Ileum

Ascending colon
Ileocolic artery and vein
Head of pancreas
Transverse colon
Superior mesenteric artery
Superior pancreaticoduodenal artery
Superior mesenteric vein
Superior part of duodenum

Left subclavian vein
Left upper lobe of lung
Left coronary artery
Left common carotid artery
Pulmonary trunk
Ascending aorta
Brachiocephalic trunk
Trachea
Brachiocephalic trunk

Right subclavian vein
Superior vena cava
Right atrium
Right upper lobe of lung
Right middle lobe of lung
Right lower lobe of lung
Right coronary artery
Middle hepatic vein
Fissure of ligamentum teres
Right lobe of liver (anterior segment)
Left branch of hepatic artery
Right lobe of liver (medial segment) quadrate
Gallbladder
Left lobe of liver (medial segment)

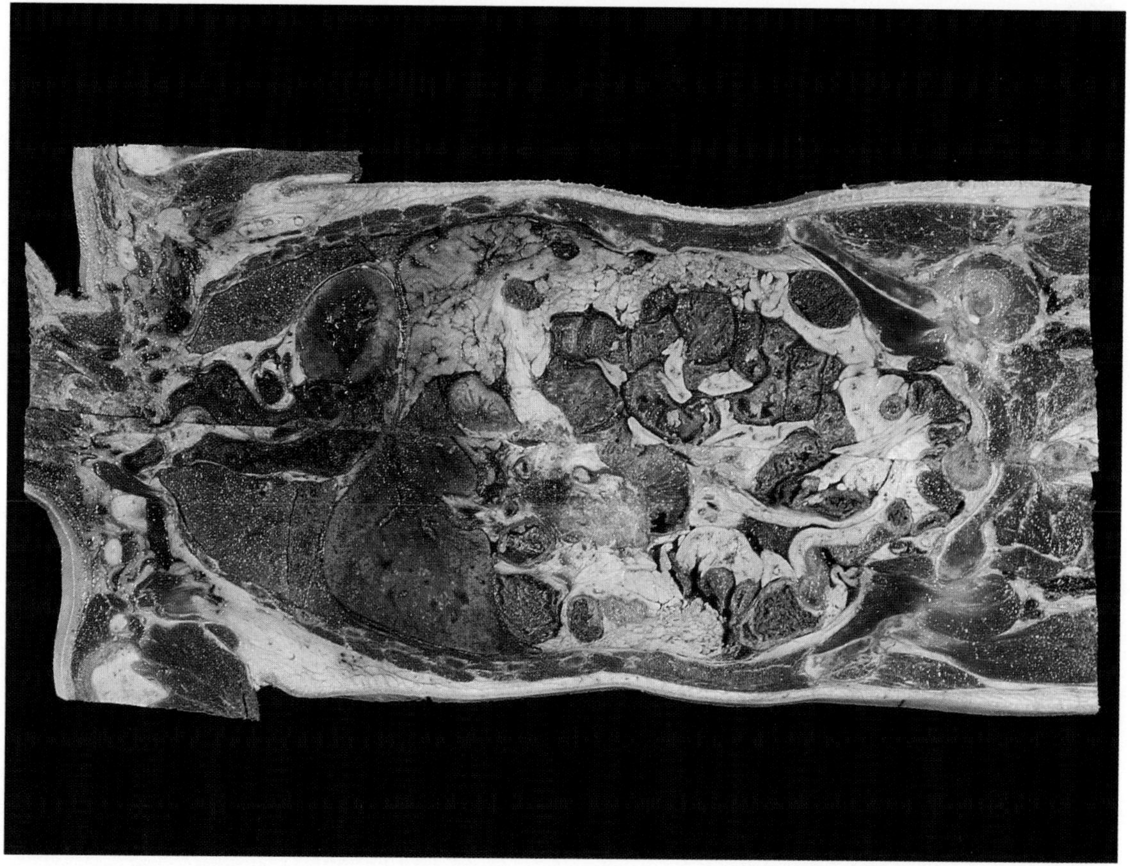

Plate 128

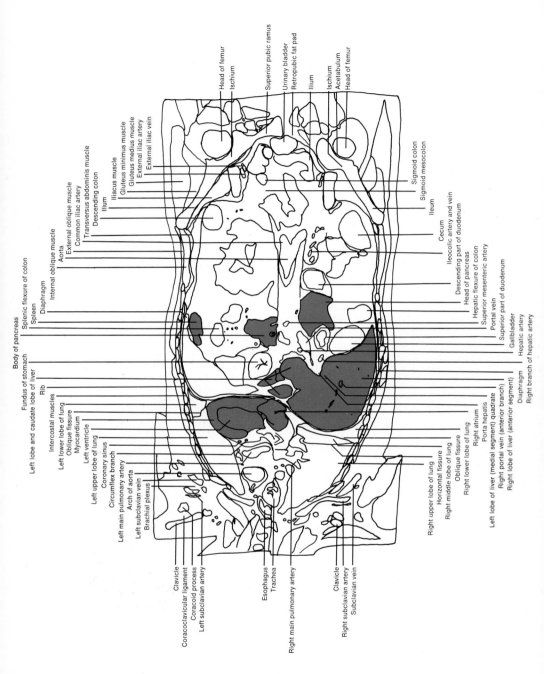

Body of pancreas
Splenic flexure of colon
Spleen
Diaphragm
Internal oblique muscle
Aorta
External oblique muscle
Common iliac artery
Transversus abdominis muscle
Descending colon
Ilium
Iliacus muscle
Gluteus minimus muscle
Gluteus medius muscle
External iliac artery
External iliac vein

Head of femur
Ischium
Superior pubic ramus
Urinary bladder
Retropubic fat pad
Ilium
Ischium
Acetabulum
Head of femur

Sigmoid colon
Sigmoid mesocolon
Ileum
Cecum
Ileocolic artery and vein
Descending part of duodenum
Head of pancreas
Hepatic flexure of colon
Superior mesenteric artery
Portal vein
Superior part of duodenum
Gallbladder
Hepatic artery
Right branch of hepatic artery

Fundus of stomach
Left lobe and caudate lobe of liver
Rib
Intercostal muscles
Left lower lobe of lung
Oblique fissure
Myocardium
Left ventricle
Left upper lobe of lung
Coronary sinus
Circumflex branch
Left main pulmonary artery
Arch of aorta
Left subclavian vein
Brachial plexus

Right upper lobe of lung
Horizontal fissure
Right middle lobe of lung
Oblique fissure
Right lower lobe of lung
Right atrium
Porta hepatis
Right portal vein (anterior branch)
Left lobe of liver (medial segment) quadrate
Diaphragm
Right lobe of liver (anterior segment)

Clavicle
Coracoclavicular ligament
Coracoid process
Left subclavian artery

Esophagus
Trachea

Right main pulmonary artery

Clavicle
Right subclavian artery
Subclavian vein

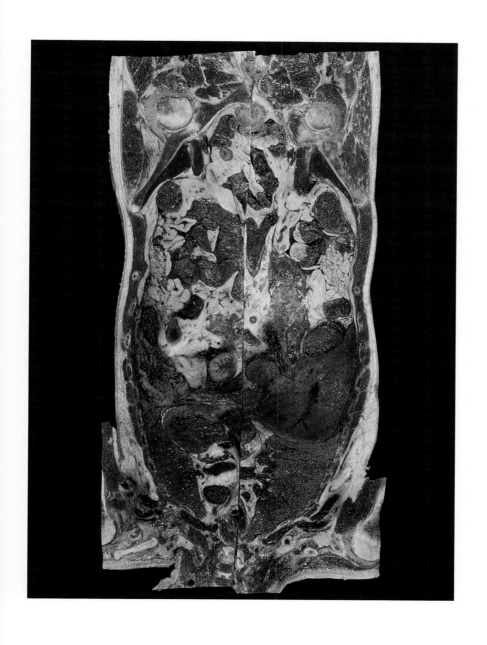

Coronal **Chest, Abdomen, and Pelvis**

Plate 129

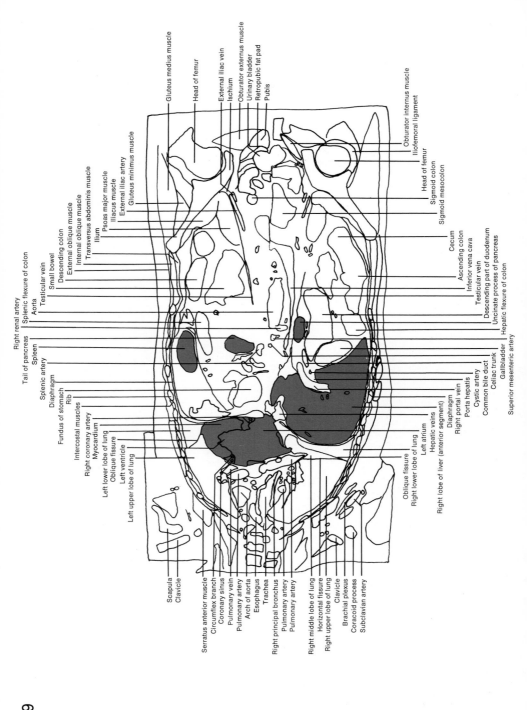
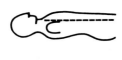

Coronal **Chest, Abdomen, and Pelvis**

Plate 130

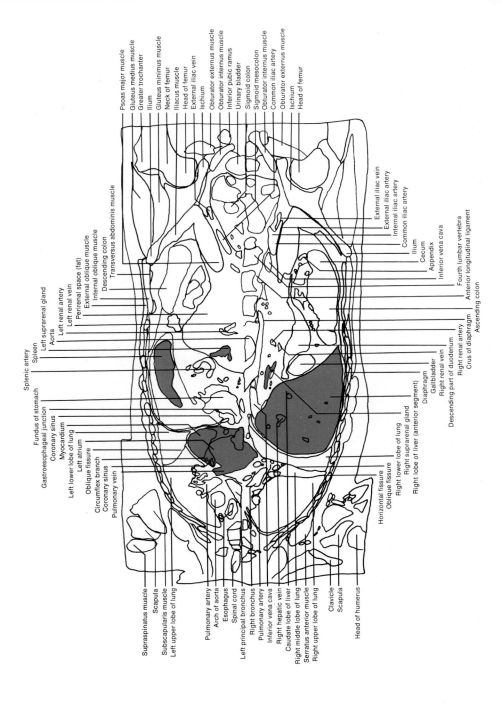

Splenic artery
Spleen
Fundus of stomach
Gastroesophageal junction
Coronary sinus
Myocardium
Left lower lobe of lung
Left atrium
Oblique fissure
Circumflex branch
Coronary sinus
Pulmonary vein

Left suprarenal gland
Aorta
Left renal artery
Left renal vein
Perirenal space (fat)
External oblique muscle
Internal oblique muscle
Descending colon
Transversus abdominis muscle

Psoas major muscle
Gluteus medius muscle
Greater trochanter
Ilium
Gluteus minimus muscle
Neck of femur
Iliacus muscle
Head of femur
External iliac vein
Ischium
Obturator externus muscle
Obturator internus muscle
Inferior pubic ramus
Urinary bladder
Sigmoid colon
Sigmoid mesocolon
Obturator internus muscle
Common iliac artery
Obturator externus muscle
Ischium
Head of femur

External iliac vein
External iliac artery
Internal iliac artery
Common iliac artery
Ilium
Cecum
Appendix
Inferior vena cava
Fourth lumbar vertebra
Anterior longitudinal ligament
Ascending colon

Horizontal fissure
Oblique fissure
Right lower lobe of lung
Right suprarenal gland
Right lobe of liver (anterior segment)
Diaphragm
Right renal vein
Right renal artery
Descending part of duodenum
Crus of diaphragm

Supraspinatus muscle
Scapula
Subscapularis muscle
Left upper lobe of lung

Pulmonary artery
Arch of aorta
Esophagus
Spinal cord
Left principal bronchus
Right bronchus
Pulmonary artery
Inferior vena cava
Right hepatic vein
Caudate lobe of liver
Right middle lobe of lung
Serratus anterior muscle
Right upper lobe of lung

Clavicle
Scapula

Head of humerus

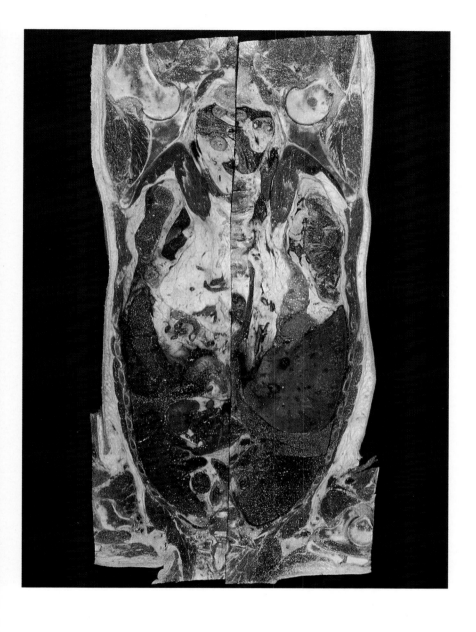

Coronal **Chest, Abdomen, and Pelvis**

Plate 131

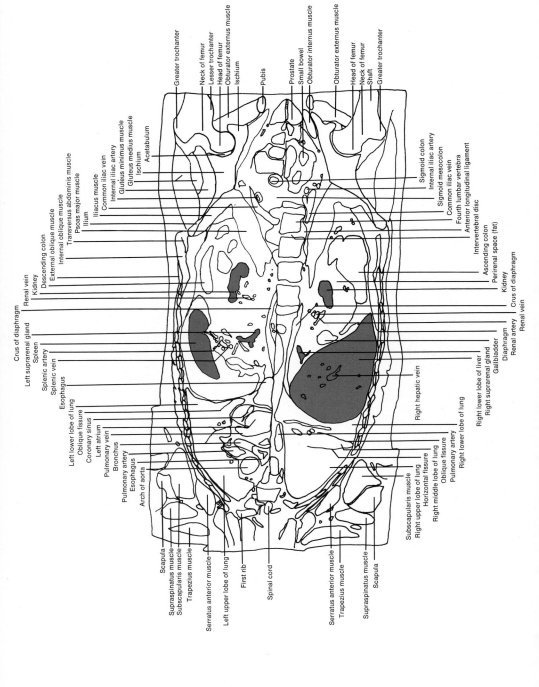

Greater trochanter
Neck of femur
Lesser trochanter
Head of femur
Obturator externus muscle
Ischium
Pubis
Prostate
Small bowel
Obturator internus muscle
Obturator externus muscle
Head of femur
Neck of femur
Shaft
Greater trochanter

Sigmoid colon
Internal iliac artery
Sigmoid mesocolon
Common iliac vein
Fourth lumbar vertebra
Anterior longitudinal ligament
Intervertebral disc
Ascending colon
Perirenal space (fat)
Kidney
Crus of diaphragm
Renal vein
Right hepatic vein
Diaphragm
Renal artery
Gallbladder
Right suprarenal gland
Right lower lobe of liver
Right lower lobe of lung
Pulmonary artery
Oblique fissure
Right middle lobe of lung
Horizontal fissure
Right upper lobe of lung
Subscapularis muscle
Scapula
Supraspinatus muscle
Trapezius muscle
Serratus anterior muscle

Acetabulum
Ischium
Gluteus medius muscle
Gluteus minimus muscle
Psoas major muscle
Common iliac artery
Internal iliac vein
Iliacus muscle
Ilium
Transversus abdominis muscle
Internal oblique muscle
External oblique muscle
Descending colon
Kidney
Renal vein
Crus of diaphragm
Left suprarenal gland
Spleen
Splenic artery
Splenic vein
Esophagus
Left lower lobe of lung
Oblique fissure
Coronary sinus
Left atrium
Pulmonary vein
Bronchus
Pulmonary artery
Esophagus
Arch of aorta
Scapula
Supraspinatus muscle
Subscapularis muscle
Trapezius muscle
Serratus anterior muscle
Left upper lobe of lung
First rib
Spinal cord

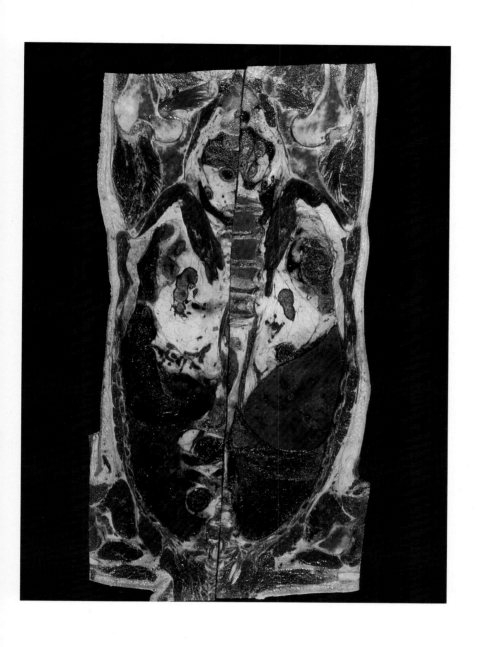

Plate 132

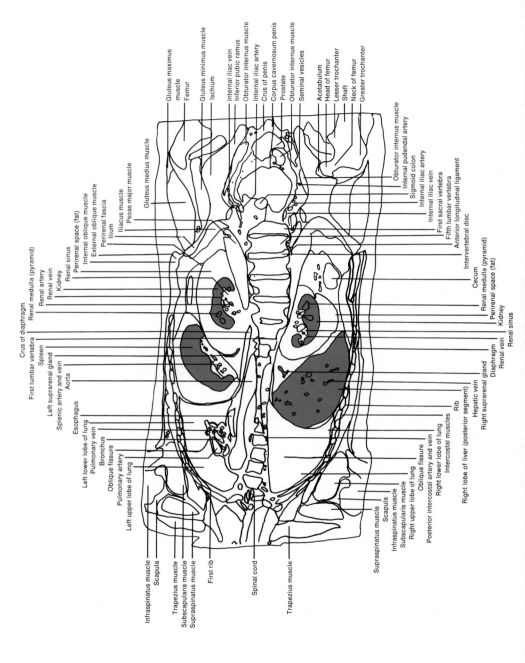

Crus of diaphragm
First lumbar vertebra
Spleen
Left suprarenal gland
Splenic artery and vein
Aorta
Esophagus
Left lower lobe of lung
Pulmonary vein
Bronchus
Oblique fissure
Pulmonary artery
Left upper lobe of lung

Renal medulla (pyramid)
Renal artery
Renal vein
Kidney
Renal sinus
Perirenal space (fat)
Internal oblique muscle
External oblique muscle
Ilium
Perirenal fascia
Iliacus muscle
Psoas major muscle
Gluteus medius muscle

Gluteus maximus
muscle
Femur
Gluteus minimus muscle
Ischium
Internal iliac vein
Inferior pubic ramus
Obturator internus muscle
Internal iliac artery
Crus of penis
Corpus cavernosum penis
Prostate
Obturator internus muscle
Seminal vesicles

Acetabulum
Head of femur
Lesser trochanter
Shaft
Neck of femur
Greater trochanter

Obturator internus muscle
Internal pudendal artery
Sigmoid colon
Internal iliac artery
Internal iliac vein
First sacral vertebra
Fifth lumbar vertebra
Anterior longitudinal ligament
Intervertebral disc
Cecum
Renal medulla (pyramid)
Perirenal space (fat)
Kidney
Renal vein
Diaphragm
Right suprarenal gland
Hepatic vein
Rib
Right lobe of liver (posterior segment)
Right lower lobe of lung
Intercostal muscles
Posterior intercostal artery and vein
Oblique fissure
Right upper lobe of lung
Subscapularis muscle
Infraspinatus muscle
Scapula
Supraspinatus muscle

Infraspinatus muscle
Scapula
Trapezius muscle
Subscapularis muscle
Supraspinatus muscle
First rib
Spinal cord
Trapezius muscle

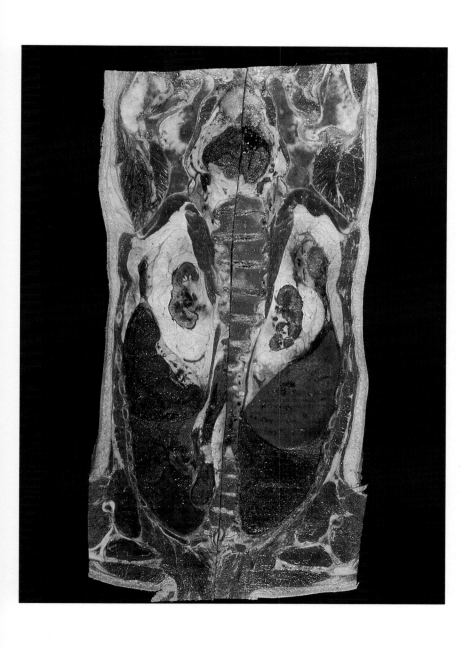

Coronal **Chest, Abdomen, and Pelvis**

Plate 133

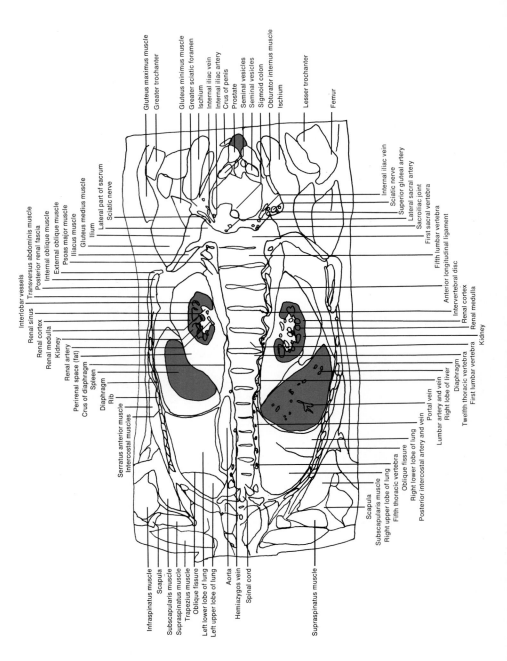

Interlobar vessels
Renal sinus
Renal cortex
Renal medulla
Kidney
Renal artery
Perirenal space (fat)
Crus of diaphragm
Spleen
Diaphragm
Rib
Serratus anterior muscle
Intercostal muscles

Transversus abdominis muscle
Posterior renal fascia
Internal oblique muscle
External oblique muscle
Psoas major muscle
Iliacus muscle
Gluteus medius muscle
Ilium
Lateral part of sacrum
Sciatic nerve

Gluteus maximus muscle
Greater trochanter
Gluteus minimus muscle
Greater sciatic foramen
Ischium
Internal iliac vein
Internal iliac artery
Crus of penis
Prostate
Seminal vesicles
Seminal vesicles
Sigmoid colon
Obturator internus muscle
Ischium
Lesser trochanter
Femur

Internal iliac vein
Sciatic nerve
Superior gluteal artery
Lateral sacral artery
Sacroiliac joint
First sacral vertebra
Fifth lumbar vertebra
Anterior longitudinal ligament
Intervertebral disc
Renal cortex
Renal medulla
Kidney

Diaphragm
Portal vein
Right lobe of liver
Lumbar artery and vein
Twelfth thoracic vertebra
First lumbar vertebra

Scapula
Subscapularis muscle
Fifth thoracic vertebra
Oblique fissure
Right lower lobe of lung
Right upper lobe of lung
Posterior intercostal artery and vein

Infraspinatus muscle
Scapula
Subscapularis muscle
Supraspinatus muscle
Trapezius muscle
Oblique fissure
Left lower lobe of lung
Left upper lobe of lung
Aorta
Hemiazygos vein
Spinal cord

Supraspinatus muscle

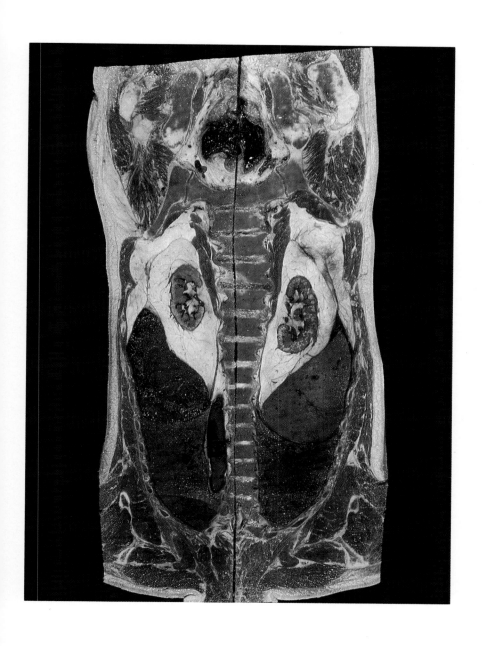

Coronal **Chest, Abdomen, and Pelvis**

Plate 134

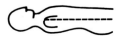

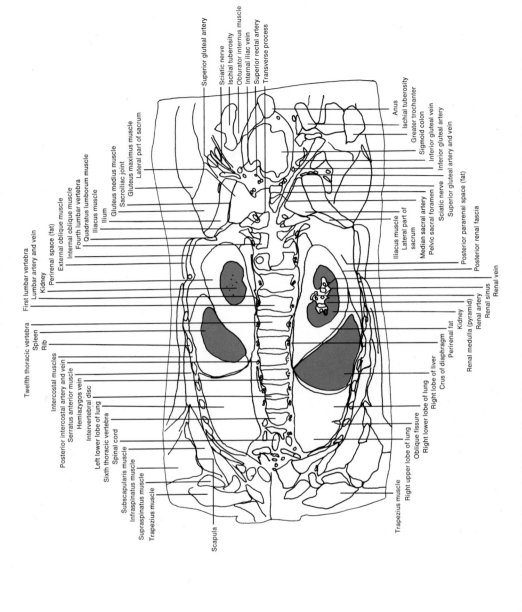

Superior gluteal artery
Sciatic nerve
Ischial tuberosity
Obturator internus muscle
Internal iliac vein
Superior rectal artery
Transverse process

Anus
Ischial tuberosity
Greater trochanter
Sigmoid colon
Inferior gluteal vein
Inferior gluteal artery
Superior gluteal artery and vein
Lateral part of sacrum

Iliacus muscle
Lateral part of sacrum
Median sacral artery
Pelvic sacral foramen
Sciatic nerve
Superior gluteal artery
Posterior pararenal space (fat)
Posterior renal fascia
Renal vein

First lumbar vertebra
Lumbar artery and vein
Kidney
Perirenal space (fat)
External oblique muscle
Internal oblique muscle
Fourth lumbar vertebra
Quadratus lumborum muscle
Iliacus muscle
Ilium
Gluteus medius muscle
Sacroiliac joint
Gluteus maximus muscle
Lateral part of sacrum

Twelfth thoracic vertebra
Spleen
Rib
Intercostal muscles
Posterior intercostal artery and vein
Serratus anterior muscle
Hemiazygos vein
Intervertebral disc
Left lower lobe of lung
Sixth thoracic vertebra
Spinal cord
Subscapularis muscle
Infraspinatus muscle
Supraspinatus muscle
Trapezius muscle

Scapula

Trapezius muscle
Right upper lobe of lung
Oblique fissure
Right lower lobe of lung
Right lobe of liver
Crus of diaphragm
Perirenal fat
Kidney
Renal artery
Renal sinus
Renal medulla (pyramid)

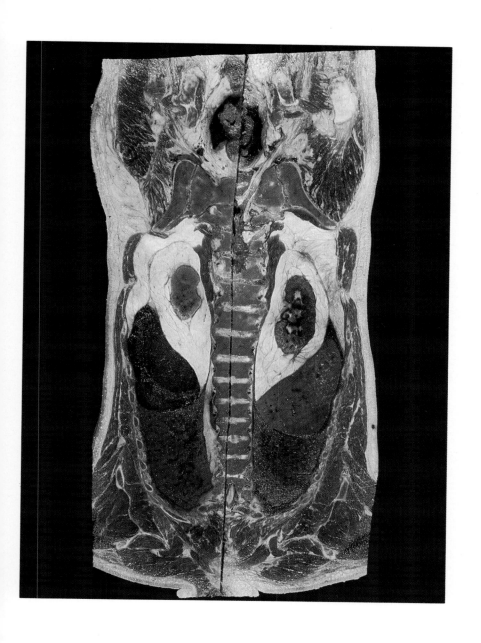

Coronal **Chest, Abdomen, and Pelvis**

Plate 135

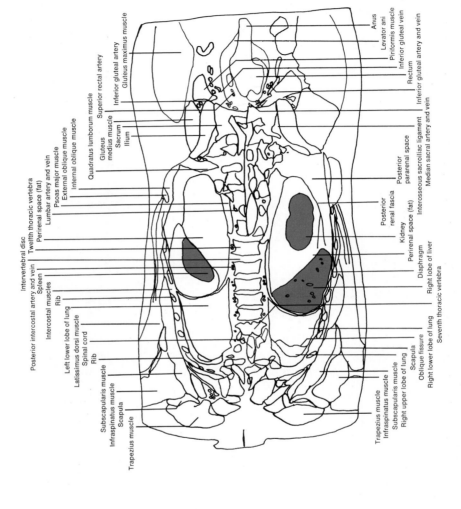

Intervertebral disc
Posterior intercostal artery and vein   Twelfth thoracic vertebra
Spleen   Perirenal space (fat)
Intercostal muscles   Lumbar artery and vein
Rib   Psoas major muscle
Left lower lobe of lung   External oblique muscle
Latissimus dorsi muscle   Internal oblique muscle
Spinal cord   Quadratus lumborum muscle
Rib   Superior rectal artery
Subscapularis muscle   Gluteus
Infraspinatus muscle   medius muscle   Inferior gluteal artery
Scapula   Sacrum   Gluteus maximus muscle
Trapezius muscle   Ilium

Anus
Levator ani
Piriformis muscle
Inferior gluteal vein
Rectum
Inferior gluteal artery and vein
Median sacral artery and vein
Interosseous sacroiliac ligament
Posterior
pararenal space
Posterior
renal fascia
Kidney
Perirenal space (fat)
Diaphragm
Right lobe of liver
Seventh thoracic vertebra

Trapezius muscle
Infraspinatus muscle
Subscapularis muscle
Right upper lobe of lung
Scapula
Oblique fissure
Right lower lobe of lung

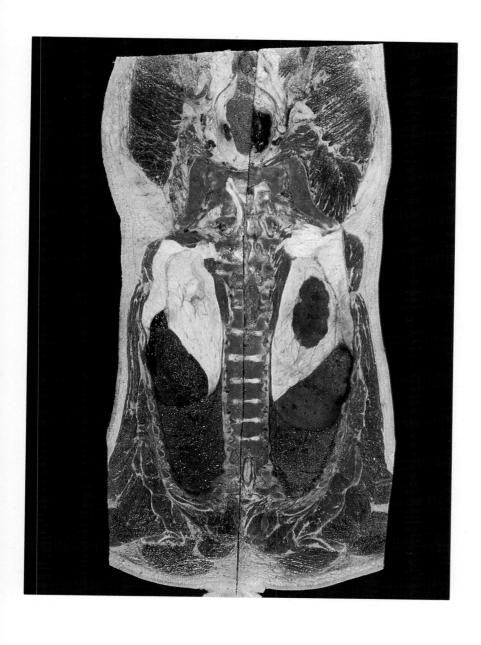

Plate 136

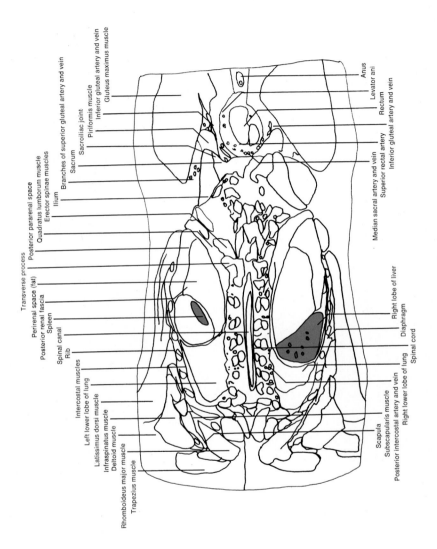

Transverse process
Posterior pararenal space
Quadratus lumborum muscle
Erector spinae muscles
Ilium
Branches of superior gluteal artery and vein
Sacrum
Sacroiliac joint
Piriformis muscle
Inferior gluteal artery and vein
Gluteus maximus muscle

Anus
Levator ani
Rectum
Inferior gluteal artery and vein
Superior rectal artery
Median sacral artery and vein

Perirenal space (fat)
Posterior renal fascia
Spleen
Spinal canal
Rib

Right lobe of liver
Diaphragm
Spinal cord

Intercostal muscles
Left lower lobe of lung
Latissimus dorsi muscle
Infraspinatus muscle
Deltoid muscle
Rhomboideus major muscle
Trapezius muscle

Scapula
Subscapularis muscle
Posterior intercostal artery and vein
Right lower lobe of lung

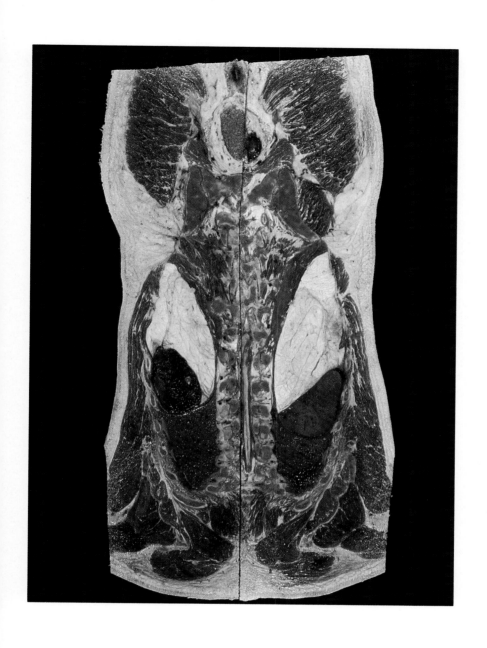

Coronal **Chest, Abdomen, and Pelvis**

Plate 137

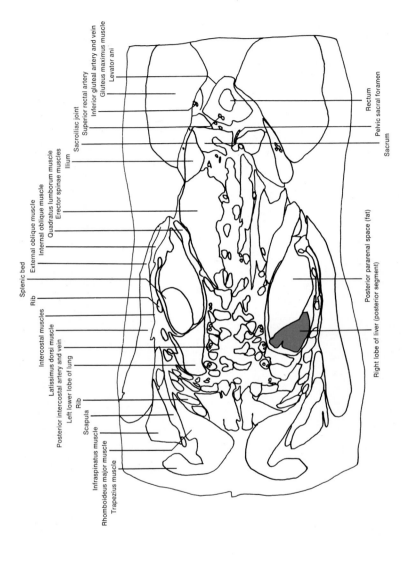

- Splenic bed
- Rib
- External oblique muscle
- Internal oblique muscle
- Quadratus lumborum muscle
- Erector spinae muscles
- Ilium
- Sacroiliac joint
- Superior rectal artery
- Inferior gluteal artery and vein
- Gluteus maximus muscle
- Levator ani

- Intercostal muscles
- Latissimus dorsi muscle
- Posterior intercostal artery and vein
- Left lower lobe of lung
- Rib
- Scapula
- Infraspinatus muscle
- Rhomboideus major muscle
- Trapezius muscle

- Rectum
- Pelvic sacral foramen
- Sacrum

- Posterior pararenal space (fat)
- Right lobe of liver (posterior segment)

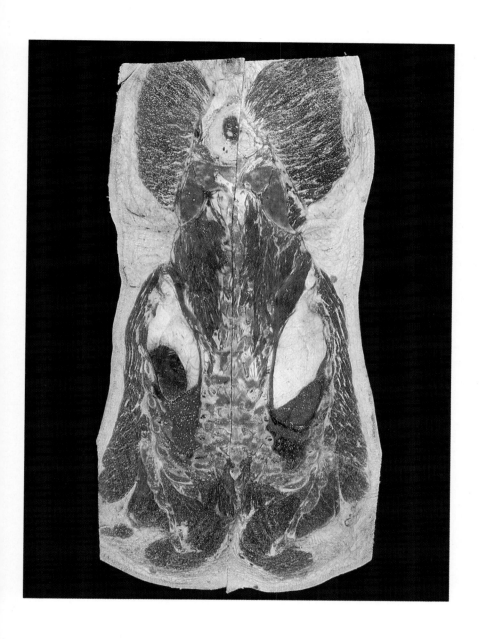

Coronal **Chest, Abdomen, and Pelvis**

Plate 138

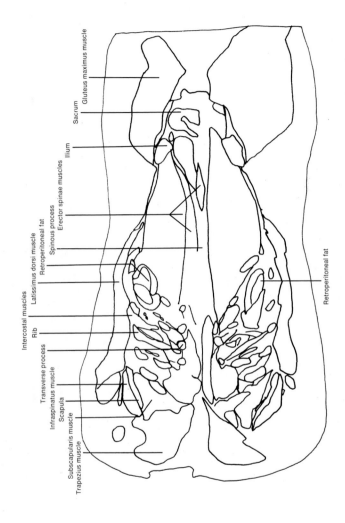

Gluteus maximus muscle

Sacrum

Ilium

Erector spinae muscles

Spinous process

Retroperitoneal fat

Latissimus dorsi muscle

Intercostal muscles

Rib

Transverse process

Infraspinatus muscle

Scapula

Subscapularis muscle

Trapezius muscle

Retroperitoneal fat

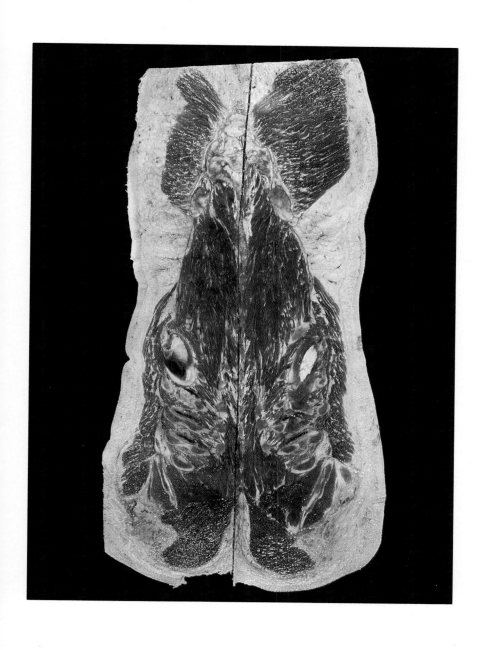

Coronal **Chest, Abdomen, and Pelvis**

INDEX

305